JOURNEY OF HEALING
Finding Healing & Hope After Abortion

Myrtzie Levell

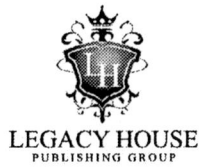

LEGACY HOUSE
PUBLISHING GROUP

Published in Mount Dora, Florida, by Legacy House Publishing Group.

www.LegacyHousePublishingGroup.net

This title may be available for purchase in bulk for educational, fund-raising or ministry use. For information, please e-mail Info@MyrtzieLevell.com

Unless otherwise noted, Scripture quotations are taken from the King James Version.

ISBN: 978-0-9906701-3-1

DEDICATION

I dedicate this book to all the babies lost through abortion, and to the mothers and fathers who haven't had the chance to mourn for them.

To my two babies in Heaven, Alicia and Thomas --- I have mourned your loss and know I will see and hold you both in Heaven. Until then I will share my story to help others find healing and hope.

To my husband and my three daughters who walked on this journey of healing with me and have given me their love and support throughout the years, thank you.

SPECIAL THANKS

I want to thank my Lord and Savior for His never ending love and His REDEMPTION. He changed my life and set me free from the bondage I was in for so long. He taught me about His truth and called me to help other women and men find healing and hope after an abortion.

Thank you to my husband, Tim, for all his love and support, and my three daughters, Jennifer, Crystal and Sheri for always loving and encouraging me along the way. Thank you for always being there. I love and appreciate you all.

Thank you to Cindy Fitzgibbon for being my right hand. You have been the help and support that I needed to help this ministry grow and put this book together. You have such passion to share your healing with others --- and you do it in such a loving and caring way. Thank you, Cindy, for all your help. I feel so honored to have you as my assistant and my friend.

Thank you to Ellie Suarez for being my left hand. You have been such a blessing in my life. Your light inside you shines so bright. Thank you for helping put the final touches on this book together. You are so passionate for this ministry. Thank you for sharing your journey of healing with everyone you come in contact with. Thank you for working for the Kingdom. I couldn't be more proud of you. I feel so privileged to have you as part of our team and to call you friend.

Thank you to Melanie Craig for proofreading this book, and all the wonderful and courageous women who have shared their personal journey of healing stories. I know God will use these testimonies to change people's lives, touch their hearts and encourage them to take the first step to begin their own journey of healing.

CONTENTS

FOREWORD

Tracee Jones

When I first reviewed the manuscript for a curriculum called First Steps Journey of Healing for Post Abortion Recovery, I quickly recognized the need for its author, Myrtzie Levell, to publish a book that heralded the stories of women who have experienced the pain of abortion, survived its aftermath and found the redemption and peace that can only be found through discovering Christ's grace and forgiveness ---- while at the same time giving women who have had an abortion(s) hope and inspiration.

These are stories you'll never see on the news, but exist nonetheless. Stories of women who have overcome their past and become beacons of light for hundreds of thousands of women.

In a society where 1 in 4 women who sit on the church pews have either experienced or been affected by abortion, it's high time that someone with the revelation and wisdom that God has given Myrtzie Levell and the brave women who share their story in this book be heard.

If this book has come into your hands and you have unresolved issues surrounding your abortion or feel like your past keeps pulling you in, I encourage you to read this book and follow the steps these women took to find wholeness and freedom from the past.

If you are pregnant and thinking about having an abortion, I encourage you to read this book in its entirety before making your final decision. Learning from the experience of others is sometimes the best guidance you can find when facing a major decision that can impact your life forever. If you need more information or are still unsure, there are telephone numbers in the back of this book of people who can answer any questions you have about the abortion process and your options.

Last but not least, if you are a parent of a young child, I challenge you to be proactive and get a copy of this book to give to your children when they are 12 or 13 years old --- and talk to them about it. Tell them you're going to keep it on the bookcase (or some other location), so that if they ever find themselves in a situation where they don't know what to do –and they feel like they can't come and talk to you about it --- they have a safe place to make an informed decision and get the help they need. As parents, sometimes we are not equipped to navigate our children through the challenges they will encounter, and it's ok. Your role as a parent is to point them in the direction of those who ARE equipped to help them, and by doing this, you will have done your job.

If you have teenagers or college age students, don't assume they will never be in a position where they must decide whether or not to have an abortion. Get them a copy of this book, ask them to read it and make time to talk with them about it. If you are uncomfortable talking with them about it, ask them to read it and leave the book somewhere they can have access to it if they ever need it.

I intend to buy a copy of this book for my children and I encourage you to do the same. As you read this book, I pray you will be blessed and encouraged by the transparency and wisdom found within its pages.

God's blessings & strength to you my friend,
Tracee Jones
Vice President
Legacy House Publishing Group

THE POWER OF CHOICE

There are many reasons a woman can find herself in a crisis pregnancy. Crisis pregnancies show no discrimination. It can happen to anyone --- no matter where you are from, how much money you make, or the color of your skin.

For whatever reason when a woman finds herself in an unplanned pregnancy, there is one thing that is certain. She will have to make a choice about what to do about the pregnancy. Unfortunately, when it comes to unplanned pregnancy, the choice is usually covered in fear. When we make a choice in the midst of fear, most of the time it will be the WRONG one.

I like to compare it to someone drowning. Imagine a woman who has floated too far out in the water. She can't touch the bottom. She doesn't know how to swim. She's in a panic, and just knows that she is going to die. She's thrashing wildly to stay on top of the water, because she knows if she starts to sink, she will never come up. Then someone comes along to save her. As the person gets close to her, she starts thrashing wildly and grabbing onto the person. As a result, they both end up drowning.

For this woman, the fear of drowning was so overwhelming that it caused her to make a choice that was fatal. Instead of allowing her rescuer to take hold of her and trust him to get her to safety, she panicked and tried to handle it her way. The result was disastrous.

We act the same way a lot of times when we are scared. Instead of taking a deep breath and trusting God to guide us through tumultuous times, we try to fix the problem our way. In the real life testimonies that you are about to read (mine included) you will see that their way did not work. It ONLY led to drowning in depression and low self-esteem.

Over 22 years ago I came to the Pregnancy Center because I was dealing with the aftermath of my two abortions. I got to experience God's redemption and He restored my brokenness. Since that time, God has used me to minister to thousands of men and women who were either thinking about abortion or had an abortion. I have worked at the Pregnancy Center for 20 years, I have gained useful information which can help you.

Women choose abortion because they are trying to solve their problem. When I went to the abortion clinic I truly thought I was solving my problem. Nobody would find out; problem solved. But it doesn't work out that way.

Abortion opens the door to many more problems such as anger, regret, shame, numbness, loneliness, grief, anguish, despair anxiety, and punishing behaviors such as eating disorders, alcoholism, drug addiction, cutting, altered femininity, damaged mothering, isolation, relationship changes, sleeping disorders, sexual dysfunction and secrecy.

These are common issues experienced in the aftermath of abortion. It is also very common for a girl to get pregnant again after one year. This is called the atonement baby (the makeup baby).

Abortion will become a deep dark secret you will carry in your heart. You will not want to let the secret out. A lot of times it stays dormant for years. This is called denial. Here's what happens. You choose to have an abortion. After it's over, you have to move forward with your life, so you shove it down deep inside and put fake smile on your face so no one will know you are dying on the inside. This is also called a defense mechanism.

When something traumatic happens, you go into denial or the numbing stage where you do not feel anything --- happy or sad. You are just going through the motions trying to make it through each day.

Eventually something will trigger the memories and the feelings you have shoved down. It might be the anniversary date of the abortion or the anniversary date of when your baby would have been born. It could be a smell or a sound. It could even be something such as hitting a brick wall. For instance, you could try to develop a close relationship with God, but as you start getting closer, your abortion slaps you in your face with thoughts like, "Remember what you did? You had an abortion. How could God love you or forgive you for that?"

When it comes to the choice of abortion, you could keep this deep dark secret and go to church every Sunday ---- singing praises to God while at the same time trying to earn your way back into God's grace. The longer you are quiet, the longer you will be in agony. Break the silence and call out to God. He is waiting for you to reach out to Him. He and His Word will embrace you and give you rest.

There is a passage in His Word that described exactly how I was feeling. It was written by King David, who had a special way with words. When I read this scripture, I could relate so much. Read the following passage and see if you can relate as well.

Psalm 38:3-11(CEB)

> *3 There's nothing in my body that isn't broken*
> *because of your rage;*
> *there's no health in my bones*
> *because of my sin.*
> *4 My wrongdoings are stacked higher than my head;*
> *they are a weight that's way too heavy for me.*
> *5 My wounds reek; they are all infected*
> *because of my stupidity.*
> *6 I am hunched over, completely down;*
> *I wander around all day long, sad.*

⁷ My insides are burning up;
*   there's nothing in my body that isn't broken.*
⁸ I'm worn out, completely crushed;
*   I groan because of my miserable heart.*
⁹ Everything I long for is laid out before you, my Lord;
*   my sighs aren't hidden from you.*
¹⁰ My heart pounds; my strength abandons me.
*   Even the light of my eyes is gone.*
¹¹ My loved ones and friends keep their distance
*   from me in my sickness;*
*   those who were near me now stay far away.*

When I read these verses I couldn't believe that David was feeling the same way I felt. Because of my sins, I was broken. The weight was just too heavy to bear. What David is describing so descriptively is depression. Can you relate to how he was feeling? I remember walking around with my head held low because I had shame in my heart. I remember feeling like I was dying inside in spite of the fake smile I had on the outside. I remember being worn out and ready to give up. Can you remember a time when you felt like you just wanted to give up? Don't give up. Keep reading. You are not alone. There are many others who have been where you are and found healing and hope.

This book is about the personal journey to healing to ten women who took the journey from guilt to gladness. As you read their stories, you will see that either they were in a crisis pregnancy or someone they loved was in a crisis pregnancy. As they share the intimate details of their lives, you will see how they made their decisions, as well as how and why they decided to choose abortion.

As you walk with them on their journey, you will feel the pain of the aftermath they went through after their choice to abort. Lastly, you will see how God called each of them to take the first step on their journey of healing.

As you read their stories, see if you can relate to their process. Don't be surprised if you discover that there are many similarities between their experiences (which you will hear me refer to as aftermath or aftermath experiences) and what you have experienced. Even though you will see similarities between your story and theirs, you will find that each experienced unique consequences to the choices they made --- just as you do.

As you read their stories of struggle and aftermath to victory, reflect on your own story. If you can relate to any of the following: a lump in your throat and fighting back tears when the word abortion is mentioned .....if you experience depression or anxiety around the anniversary date of your abortion....if the smell of antiseptic or the sound of a vacuum causes you to have flashbacks....if you experience nightmares of crying babies.... if you look at other children and wonder if that is how old your child would be....if whenever you are in a church service (and the sermon is on abortion), your heart begins to race, your hands begin to sweat, you feel like you have a big neon sign on your forehead flashing, "I had an abortion! I had an abortion!".... then you are ready to take the first step on your own journey of healing.

When you read the stories of these courageous women, I am praying that they bring you hope and encourage you to start YOUR journey of healing.

Sandy's Journey of Healing
A Gift from God Handled Incredibly Wrong

*A*ll of 1985 my husband and I were in a dream come true life – living in Melbourne, Australia and working with a company we had been with for 19 years. Coming back to the U.S. was also wonderful because we missed our family.

In the summer of 1986 a precious young friend came to ask my opinion regarding a situation she was in. She was pregnant and the father of the baby was a drug dealer whom she really disliked. She did not want him to know about the pregnancy. She wanted him out of her life. She asked me the question, "Do you think abortion is the answer?"

Although this is still so painful to share, I am going to be very transparent with you. There should have been no hesitation on my part. I was a Christian, married mother of two. I responded by asking her to find out more about an abortion before a decision was made. At that time, I really did not know about the consequences associated with abortion. I thought it would be a simple routine procedure.

Also, because she was a close friend, I knew that if she became a single mother, it would impact my life. I would have to be there for her and my husband and I were in the middle of changing our lifestyle. With this in mind, I gave her the most selfish answer. Instead of telling her that abortion was not the answer and I would be there for her, I asked her to find out more about the abortion procedure.

Her findings surprised me. She was told that based on how far along in her pregnancy she was, it was not yet a baby and if she hurried --- before the week was over --- it would be okay to have an abortion. I think she and I knew all along what the truth was, but had already made up our minds. When my friend asked if the abortion would hurt, she was told that for $50 more they could sedate her. I agreed to help her with this cost.

There were many girls in the lobby of the abortion clinic that morning. Most of them were relaxed and unconcerned. Some were even laughing. I remember thinking, "If I felt we were doing nothing wrong, why am I so uncomfortable?"

While my young friend checked in, I waited in the lobby. She looked so scared. I wanted to comfort her, but I was not allowed in the back abortion rooms. After seemingly hours had passed, my friend came into the lobby. We both had a sense of relief it was all over.

We left without exchanging any words, anxious to leave this whole experience behind. We actually went to lunch although neither of us was hungry. She stayed in our home for several days afterwards. It was about four years later before we ever brought it up again. Denial can last for decades.

The only reason the subject was brought up again, is because an opening became available at the Pregnancy Center for a director. The original director was going into the mission field to Africa. I felt qualified based on my experience in Evangelism Explosion and also my husband and I managed 30 managers for Tupperware in Savannah, Georgia. Most importantly, I felt God's calling on my life and began dreaming about the wonderful volunteers and how we could affect the lives of women who needed guidance in an unplanned pregnancy.

The memories began to bubble up. I had already started the process of learning about abortion and was deeply pained by the counsel I had given my friend many years before. The basic fact that life begins at conception devastated me. I didn't have to read a library of books for God to break my heart.

God in His Grace allowed me to be hired as the director of the Pregnancy Center. I felt I could just put the past behind me, but I couldn't. I began crying at unusual times over really nothing. It was then I knew I needed healing from my past. The director before me had been inspired by the Holy Spirit to write a post abortion Bible Study called First Steps to help the women of our church heal from abortion.

First Steps already had some groups started when I got there. At first I was just going to go to observe. My husband's discernment kicked in really fast and he said the girls would see right through that. He felt I needed to go into the group like the others who were in need of post abortion healing.

Mine was so painful because I influenced a sweet friend to abort her baby. A few years later, she went through the Bible Study too. There is only one place to seek healing and that is through God. He was faithful. He often uses our pain for His Glory but only when He sees our heart is focused on Him. I then saw that God was going to use my experience to help others make the right decision with God's precious gift of pregnancy and the life of a baby.

Minelly's Journey of Healing
Filled with God's Love

*I*t's not by chance that you've come across this book of stories. There's a reason why you're reading this book. Maybe someone you know (or you yourself) has had a similar experience. Whatever the condition may be, may you find peace and strength as you continue to read.

Years have passed, and here I am reluctantly writing about my past, reluctant mostly because I don't want to remember, but also because I have already given my past to the Lord. My purpose in telling my story is to help anyone who may have experienced one of life's tragic blows with the power to paralyze our very core and spirit ---in such a way that the only thing that can release us from the bondage of guilt and regret would be found in the arms of our Savior.

Many years ago, I fell out of grace with my Heavenly Father and had an abortion (three to be exact). As I look back, I wonder how I could have been so selfish and cruel to myself and to my unborn children. I can only credit lack of knowledge and understanding for life and God at the time.

I was in a new country without a mother, father and close relatives. I was seeking to better my circumstances and had migrated to the United States in search of my hopes and dreams. Neither prevailed…

After being here and working diligently to suppress the loneliness of being away from home and family, I met a man at a bus stop one day. After spending six months together, I knew that he wasn't the person that I wanted to spend the rest of my life with because he was an abusive and controlling person.

However, after six months, I became pregnant and was feeling more alone, confused, frustrated, scared and hurt than ever because my boyfriend wanted me to have an abortion. He said that he was not ready for kids and that if I cared about him I would have the abortion. He also said that he would leave me if I didn't. Although I didn't think I would spend the rest of my life with him, I also didn't want to be by myself and I didn't know anyone in this country except for co- workers. I didn't know what to do.

I did not have any of the feelings you'd expect. When we see people on TV announce that they're pregnant, they get hugs and kisses and friends and family start planning the baby shower and asking whether they want a boy or a girl. They start choosing names and the father of the baby is beside himself with joy and happiness. Nope! It sure didn't feel like that.

Instead two weeks later (after being pressured for days and completely neglected by him), I found myself in a doctor's office, in a secluded part of town -- sitting on a cold bench and looking down at the floor --- because I didn't want anyone to see me and pass judgment on me.

After the abortion, I thought it was over, but I had only made a temporary fix to a permanent scar on my life --- not just physically, but also emotionally. It was the beginning of a catastrophic journey that changed the course of my entire life and who I was.

When I had the abortion, I thought I had emptied myself of my burden. Having the abortion only got rid of what was physically inside me. I had emptied myself only to be filled with something else that would continue to grow inside me. I just couldn't see it until many years later, after I had been transformed into something other than what I was supposed to be.

After my first abortion, I thought everything would be fine and life would go back to normal. A couple of days went by the same as any other. But as time continued, I didn't feel too happy. I couldn't sleep and was without peace and without joy.

Not having anyone to confide in made it even more difficult. I didn't have any family members here in this country and not many people I could call friends. I was alone. Although my boyfriend was there, I felt alone. I couldn't talk to him about my feelings because he never considered the fetus to be a living being anyway. Back then, I had not realized that my baby was a spirit even before it came to be inside me. Ephesians 1:4 says:

> *"For He chose us in Him before the creation of the world to be holy and blameless in His sight..."*

God knew me and my kids before the foundation of the world! Everything from whom he or she would look like, his or her traits and characteristics including their smile and eye color were already thought of by our Heavenly Father. I didn't know these things back then. No one told me.

So, I went back to work. I returned to my daily routine. At first, things seemed to be getting better, but as time went by I was beginning to notice changes in me ---- little things at first. I couldn't look at people's babies. I didn't want to be around happy pregnant people and slowly I began resenting my boyfriend. Time passed and once again I became pregnant. The same scenario occurred. He said if I loved him, I would get an abortion and he would leave me if I didn't. This time I called his bluff, and he left. I was devastated and beside myself -- not knowing how I would handle this situation alone. I couldn't eat or sleep, and I began to perform poorly on my job. I felt sick every day and vomited a lot in the mornings.

I had no one now --- not even my boyfriend. I was beginning to take a lot of time off from work due to morning sickness, and my paychecks were not enough to cover my rent and utilities. Eventually my boss indicated that he would have to replace me, so I went and aborted my child the second time.

My boyfriend started coming around again. I didn't know how to feel --- no emotions, just numbness now. I knew that inside I was changing. I had begun living in fear that he would leave again and he threatened me with leaving constantly so I did what he did, went where he went and did as he said. I felt like I couldn't function on my own anymore. I didn't want to think. I could only function if someone told me what to do. I began to feel as if I couldn't make my own decisions anymore, so I let someone else do it for me, and began to slowly retreat within myself.

As time passed I started using birth control pills and trying different birth control methods. I became pregnant a third time. My boyfriend told me the baby would be deformed because of all the birth control pills I had taken, and I had to abort it. The doctor confirmed what he said, so I decided to have a third abortion.

Jesus said, "Know the truth and the truth will set you free." I didn't know the truth of what I was doing to my soul, my spirit or my unborn children. At this point I had lost all sense of myself. I became numb to feelings and lived in an abusive relationship thinking that I deserved whatever punishment I got for this disobedience.

This went on for years --- only functioning to please my boyfriend. I had no life, no feelings for myself, and didn't want anything for myself. I felt worthless, and of course, my boyfriend would tell me I was worthless. He would tell me that no one would want me after the things I had done.

Months and months went by, but it didn't matter. I felt so numb. I couldn't feel anything; it seemed as though everything was taken from inside me --- my heart, my womb, my soul.

I hated my boyfriend. I hated myself for allowing such a thing to happen to me. I had ended my children's lives before they had a chance in this world. I didn't know how much God loved me or how much love I had to give my kids.

To explain how the abortions affected my life is a bit hard because the effects did not happen overnight, but strung out for years. It gradually ate away at my core filling me with regret, hopelessness, fear and anger. It was like a great dark hole was inside of me. The thought of not being able to hold my kids, kiss them, hug them and love them was an unending torture.

I had given up the wonderful opportunity and privilege to see the faces of my babies, give them a name, dress them, hug them and love them. I didn't know God would have provided. It's a promise He had made a long time ago....to never leave us nor forsake us. One thing sure about God is that He cannot lie and cannot deny Himself.

Many years after my abortions, I married my boyfriend because I felt I didn't deserve anyone better. I felt that I needed to be punished for the things I had done. I had two kids afterwards and they are the world to me. I never forgot the ones I had given up. It tore at my very core every day, especially when I looked at my son. I cried a lot thinking about what the others would've looked like, what names I would have given them and how much older they would've been. My son would have had older siblings here to play with. Instead, he and I were left alone most of the time while my husband went out partying, committing adultery and drinking until he was sometimes unconscious.

One day I was in church when the pastor preached a sermon on abortion. I felt like melting into the cracks of the church floor, but I felt God saying "that is enough". I had to face my past and overcome the hurt and pain and move on. If I was to have a future and raise my kids and give them a good future, I had to face this. I wanted to leave during the sermon, but I couldn't, because I thought that people would look at me and be able to tell what I did all those years ago. Also, my kids were with me and I didn't want them asking questions.

The pastor showed me how lost I was and how much God loved me. He helped me understand that God wanted to have a relationship with me and would forgive me if I asked. He also showed me how God was waiting for me to come to Him like a daughter to a father and give my burden to Him. I didn't quite believe it at that moment but then, he said something that changed everything and almost caused me to scream out with joy. He said that my unborn children were in Heaven with God. Yes! He said that I would see them one day when I die, but the most horrendous thing was that I might not be able to be with them if I didn't get right with God.

I knew how great my sin was. I was afraid to come to God, but the pastor explained that if we confessed our sins to God He would forgive us and cleanse us, and we then would become a new creation in Christ. I needed to be a new creature, I didn't like the one I was.

The pastor also told about the pregnancy center and how I could receive counseling and have someone pray with me and help me overcome the tribulation in my life. I went to the center, and as time passed I learned so many wonderful things about God from very caring and loving people. I learned how I would get a second chance to live a better life as a new creation and how my past sins would be wiped away and forgotten by God and whenever He looked upon me, He would see me as He sees His wonderful son, Christ ---righteous and blameless. I also learned I could come and lay my burdens upon Him and He would carry them away and give me rest, peace, and even a chance to see and be with my unborn children. Hallelujah! Hallelujah!

Isn't God wonderful? Way back then when I was sinning so badly, He was planning and preparing to turn those sinful things I had done into good things for me one day in the future. Who can do that?! No one!

You see, way back then, while I was sitting in that doctor's office waiting to give up my unborn children, He already knew of the pain, the hurt, the anger, the frustration and turmoil my life would have to endure because of the mistakes I was about to make. No one sat there with me to tell me these things. I'm glad the pastor told me! I realize how much Jesus loves me --- to take my place in death, so I could have the opportunity to live life eternally and be with God and my children (ALL of them.)

I was about forty years old when I gave my life to Christ at the pregnancy center, and do you know the huge void and emptiness that was in the center of me? It didn't get filled right away, but as I learned about God and His love for me each time I attended a session at the center, the void gradually became smaller and smaller. Now I am filled with God's love, a love I know is peaceful and comforting. Now that's love.

I think of my kids in Heaven often, but no longer with regret, but with anticipation of meeting them one day.

I felt ashamed back then, but that is what the enemy wanted me to feel, because he is a liar and a thief. He stole my kids from me by means of abortion and told me a lot of lies. He convinced me that I was worthless and I believed that lie for many, many years.

I have had two beautiful children since that time. I have had a rough marriage, not because of my kids, but because of an abusive situation. My life is not a fairy tale. I have since divorced my husband and am raising my children on my own with God's help. I'm looking to Him for my provisions, not a man. I'm looking to Him for my comfort and strength, and for help with raising my kids, and I can truly say, that although I have rough days, God always provides a way for me and my children. I lack none of the essential things we need to live and I look to Him each day for guidance and direction as my children and I continue to grow in His everlasting love.

I pray my story has comforted you in some way as you realize (as I have) that our God is the everlasting supreme creator of the heavens and earth and His written words to us shall never fail us. As He has said, "Heaven and Earth shall pass away, but His words will remain everlasting". This is what I hold on to every day, as He sees me through day after precious day, and I look forward to a blessed future.

May God bless and keep you.

Cindy's Journey of Healing
Rescued by His Love

*M*y name is Cindy, and I thank God for the blessing of being a part of First Steps Ministry since 2007. I will never forget the courage needed to take my first step to begin my journey of healing.

This is the story of my journey. It is a sacred testimony of what God does in a human heart. It is a story about the redemption, love, and restoration found only in Jesus Christ. He has grown me in His truth and grace with each step I have taken through Him. And I am still in the making, for His transformation is not an event, but a process. In sharing my story with you, I pray your heart will be drawn to know the power of His presence and hope for His healing in your life.

Lost

I still can't recall the exact date (that is how deeply I buried my pain so many years ago) but I remember I was the young age of 17. I was naïve and lost somewhere on the wrong path in life when I became pregnant. As I reflect on my time of crisis, I remember being full of fear and feeling desperately alone. At that time, all I had was my boyfriend to turn to for help, so I thought.

It was the summer going into my Senior year when I met him. Our two worlds collided, and I was quickly attracted to his charm as I allowed his world (which was very different from my own) to become my world. He seemed to really care about me, but I soon discovered it was all lies and deception.

There were so many red flags as I became emotionally involved with him. But instead of fleeing, I accepted him --- not for

31

who he was, but for who he was hoping he would change into or who I could possibly change him into. BIG MISTAKE!

Sadly at that time in my life, I had no relationship with my earthly father or Heavenly Father. I now understand how with those missing in my life, there was a void and emptiness I was trying to fill with a boy.

I was always a people pleaser, even if I was being used, and I pretended to have good self-esteem, when I really had none. From my early childhood on, I was given the nick name "Piglet". Every time they would call me this, it would make me feel fat and ugly. I believe this is where my low-self-esteem started. I became consumed with my weight and appearance. *Dad, your how cout why we don't*

I didn't realize it at the time, but my desire to please my boyfriend --- and allowing his attraction to me dictate my self-worth --- made me "his puppet". Whatever he said, I did. He *being served* didn't want me hanging out with my friends or family because they were all trying to help me see his unhealthy and harmful ways.

I already had a strained relationship with my parents, but my choice to continue seeing him made it worse. Over time, my friends, with good reason, stopped coming around as well. And then…it happened…

Being so young and naïve, I didn't fully comprehend the consequences of the choices I was making, and how dark my path had become until I became pregnant. I will never forget how afraid I was of my parents finding out. And now with no friends, I felt so alone in my deepest despair! I felt trapped!

In my despair and bondage of fear, I traded his lies for truth and I allowed my boyfriend to take control of the situation. He set up the appointment, drove me there, and paid for the procedure. As a "puppet" I followed. To this day, I can't remember a lot of the details, but I do remember being put to sleep before the procedure.

When I awoke, I remember sitting in a chair waiting to be picked up, feeling so empty and wanting it all to be over. I was so young and naïve, I still didn't fully comprehend that I had just allowed myself to make the worst decision of my life in taking my child's life through abortion. But I do remember at that moment wanting to bury all the hurt, pain, and shame deep down inside of me and never going there again. And that is exactly what I did. It became my hidden secret for the next 25 years.

Afterwards I tried to move on with my life and do better despite my hidden secret. My unhealthy relationship with my boyfriend ended a year later when I realized he wasn't going to change, and I grew weary of trying to change him.

In Isaiah 61:1-3, the Lord promises that He opens the prison to them that are bound, and He gives beauty for ashes, and the garment of praise for the spirit of despair and heaviness. Before I would experience the Lord's healing, I continued to carry "my spirit of despair and heaviness" for many more years.

On the outside you would never know the hurt I carried because I became very good at wearing a mask. But on the inside, I silently suffered with my hidden secret. When you hold that kind of hurt, pain, shame, and sin inside of you for as long as I did, sooner or later it has to come out through destructive behaviors.

For me, I already struggled with low self-esteem and my weight, but it became worse. For several years after my abortion, I struggled with sporadic eating disorders. I also struggled with depression, mood swings, anger and guilt. I never identified any of these struggles as being related to my abortion because, in my mind, that was a part of my past that I had already dealt with. I had buried deep inside and moved on.

In 1986 I met my wonderful husband John. He was raised Catholic and was going to church when I met him, so I decided to join him. I believed in God, but I didn't know Him or His Word, or have a personal relationship with Him through Jesus Christ. My mom took us to church when I was younger, but we stopped after moving to the country in 1976. I also remember going with friends during my high school years, but it had been a long time since I had gone to church consistently.

John and I decided to get married in 1989. In order for us to get married in the Catholic Church, we needed to attend an engagement weekend retreat, so we did. I wanted us to have a healthy relationship with no secrets, so at this retreat I felt led to tell him about my hidden secret.

But in order for me to be able to talk about it, I had to stay in control of my emotions and not go too deep. I remember sharing with him like it was a box that I was taking off the shelf for the first time in a long time. I knew what was deep inside, but I was only going to look in on the surface. After sharing my secret with John, I remember quickly burying it back down inside of me, hoping that would be the last time I would ever have to bring up my past again.

Years had passed. I was now happily married, and John and I wanted to have children. After years of trying, we were unable to get pregnant. I remember thinking that God was punishing me for what I had done and I was becoming very bitter and angry.

I was still clinging to the enemy's lies that I was unworthy and living with the guilt and shame of what I had done. I was unable to forgive myself. Because of this, I was still in bondage with my hidden secret and continued to carry a spirit of despair and heaviness for several more years.

Then in 1995, God blessed us with our wonderful daughter, and in 1998 our wonderful son. It was then, as I began living out my years of motherhood, that I started to realize even more what a horrible mistake I had made in choosing abortion.

Even though I was so happy to have been blessed with my son and daughter, I continued to silently suffer internally with my hidden secret. As I continued daily life masking my wound, other hurt continued to pile on top of that wound, until one day I reached my breaking point and realized I couldn't go on any longer dealing with all the hurt I felt inside, nor did I want to.

For the first time in a very long time, I reached for my Bible and read Matthew 11:28-29. Jesus said, "Come to me, all you who are weary and burdened, and I will give you rest. Take my yoke upon you and learn from me, for I am gentle and humble in heart and you will find rest for your souls."

All those years I had gone to church with John, I loved God and believed in Him, but I still didn't know Him through His Son, Jesus Christ. His words to me that night were an invitation that God knew I needed to hear. I needed that for my soul and I needed to come to Him. So I began seeking the Lord with all my heart, soul, and mind wanting to know more about Him. Over the next couple of years, I studied His word and I grew in my faith and in His grace. I grew to understand my need for a Savior's rescue and I surrendered my life to Jesus!

Rescued

From that point on, His gift of grace began changing everything….my heart, my direction and my attitude. Because I hid my secret for 25 years and was so broken on the inside from the destruction of my abortion, I was still struggling with facing my past even after surrendering my life to Jesus. But the Holy Spirit began revealing my need for healing. So as He led me to people and places, I followed.

Then finally in 2007, after 25 years of hiding my secret, God led me to First Steps, a post- abortive healing Bible Study where I began my journey of healing. I didn't realize how in bondage I was until I began to heal!

Each week we focused on God's Word and His character. His truth began to defeat the lies I chose to believe for so many years. I began to understand that God wasn't punishing me, rather He was waiting for me to turn back to Him with a repentant heart so He could restore me. I also began to understand it wasn't about me forgiving myself, but about me understanding the forgiveness of Jesus!

I learned my worth isn't in what I do, but in what Jesus already did for me, even when I didn't deserve it! He died for me so I could be rescued and redeemed! As I began to understand His truth, my broken heart full of sorrow and repentance began to experience the love, grace and forgiveness of Jesus Christ. Only through His healing and transformation could the bondage and darkness from my past sin no longer hold me. As God promised in Isaiah, He opened my prison, took away my heaviness and despair, and gave me beauty for ashes!

Because of the forgiveness and redemption of my Lord and Savior, I now understand I have a child in Heaven. Through much prayer, I have named him Timothy-Paul and I long for the day I will meet him and be able to wrap my arms around him!

October 15, 2007 was my new beginning. God wants me to remember it in place of all those dates and details I couldn't remember about my past. It is the date we held a special night of honor to remember Timothy-Paul's precious life. Because of his precious life, I now devote my life to upholding God's truth about the sanctity of life, helping others not make the same mistake I did. I have been blessed to be a part of First Steps Ministry since 2007.

Lord, Help me to have selfless faith
Heal my heart and make it clean
Open up my eyes to the things You want me to see
Show me how to love like You love me
Break my heart for what breaks Yours
Everything I am for You and Your kingdom's cause
As I walk from earth into eternity
Let me bring you glory
Help me to have selfless faith

Reflecting back on my 25 years of bondage, I see that only God could take a heart like mine --- one so broken and in bondage from the hurt of my abortion --- and restore and transform it with a passion to serve Him in this ministry!

Because of my past, my heart is passionate in wanting to help other women and men know the love, grace and forgiveness found only in Jesus Christ. He heals their hurt, pain and brokenness from abortion. I know this is God's call for my life and through His grace, love, and truth, He gives us a profound passion and drive to do something that we could never do on our own. He is full of surprises and when you surrender your life to Him, beautiful change can happen!

It wasn't long after my journey of healing began I found myself on the other side of this with a changed heart. In the fall of 2010, through God's grace, I felt the Holy Spirit leading me to join a group called 40 Days For Life.

It is a faith-based effort bringing together the body of Christ for prayer and fasting, community outreach, and a peaceful vigil to end abortion. We gathered in front of the abortion clinic, Planned Parenthood, every day for 40 days, from 7am to 7pm, to make a presence known for Christ praying and witnessing. If someone had told me five years earlier that I would one day be standing in front of an abortion clinic trying to help women choose life, I would have told them they were crazy and they didn't know me very well!

But there I was, with a changed heart, wanting to help these women know the truth before they made the same mistake I did. I started praying and crying out to God. Slowly He led me to speak to these precious women, with whom I could relate to for I once experienced their same fear and bondage.

My heart's desire was for them to hear, understand and receive that they had other options. I wanted them to know they could get help for the precious life growing inside of them and to understand God loved them so much!

We had some incredible moments of rejoicing as we talked with some of them, sharing Christ's love for them and their babies. God definitely showed us the power of His presence as we were faithful in prayer.

But God also broke my heart during those 40 days. He was showing me the things that break His heart. I know too well the deep rooted wound from an abortion, the agonizing pain and tear in your heart that burdens you night and day from the loss of life, separating you from your loving Heavenly Father who wants nothing more than for you to know Him and experience the abundant life He created you to have in Him! But instead you allow the enemy's bondage of fear and lies to overcome you and keep you in your pit of despair.

Oh, how my heart still remembers that pit! As I stood out there each day, I mourned for those women and babies. I was so completely humbled and reminded from where God had brought me. I know I am nothing without my God and Savior, His grace, His truth, and His life He gave for me. I don't ever want to forget how He rescued me and brought me out of my pit of despair with a changed heart! On our journey, He does His work in our hearts and lives through the small, faithful steps we take in Him.

My story is a sacred testimony of what God does in a human heart. It is a story about my journey of being rescued by love, redemption and restoration found only in Jesus Christ. Yes, in my past I allowed the enemy to derail my life with lies and destruction, but now my past can be used to bring God glory! Genesis 50:20 says, "You thought evil against me; but God meant it unto good, to bring to pass, as it is this day, to save much people alive." Only He could take a heart like mine, so broken and in bondage for 25 years from the hurt of my past abortion, and restore and transform it with a passion for His sanctity of life, weaving it into His story of redemption.

During the 40 Days For Life campaign, around the world 788 lives were spared from abortion. So for His glory and honor, and in honor of my precious son in Heaven, Timothy-Paul, I will continue to devote my life to sharing my story with others so they can know the hurt and destruction from abortion and the hope for rescue, redemption, healing and restoration found only in Jesus Christ! Praise God from whom all blessings flow!

Rescued by His love,
Cindy

And I thank Christ Jesus our Lord, who hath enabled me, for that he counted me faithful, putting me into the ministry; who was before a blasphemer, and a persecutor, and injurious: but I obtained mercy, because I did it ignorantly in unbelief. And the grace of our Lord was exceeding abundant with faith and love which is in Christ Jesus. This is a faithful saying, and worthy of all acceptation, that Christ Jesus came into the world to save sinners; of whom I am chief. Howbeit for this cause I obtained mercy, that in me Jesus Christ might show forth all longsuffering, for a pattern to them which should hereafter believe on Him to life everlasting. Now unto the King eternal, immortal, invisible, the only wise God, be honour and glory for ever and ever. Amen.

~ 1 Timothy 1:12-17 KJV

Ellie's Journey of Healing
Saved by Grace

*H*i, my name is Ellie and I'd like to share my testimony with you. I pray it will give you comfort in knowing you're not alone. My husband and I have known each other since before he was born. I was a year older than he so I'd wiggle around on his mommy's belly as she held me.

We were always close and we played together. I always wanted him to be my baby dolls' daddy. Sometimes he would play along. By the time we were about 10 or 11 he began to hate girls so I became his number one enemy. During the next two years I was stupid, skinny and ugly. I was devastated! Really, what girl would want to be viewed with those attributes? Thankfully that didn't last too long. By the time we entered our teens, we liked each other a lot but now sports had entered his life. He didn't have time for me anymore. At fourteen, he began to notice me again and was I excited!

My parents were extremely strict and traditional so I wasn't allowed to date or court, but because Tony's family and my family were close, my dad gave me permission to court Tony. (Now I realize that courting is a concept that we rarely practice anymore, so I'll explain it for those of you who are wondering what it is. In a nutshell, it's dating with the intent to marry ---- as opposed to just dating.) I was fifteen at the time and very excited that he would be my boyfriend. Our relationship was on and off until I was seventeen.

My dad was strict and an alcoholic, and he believed anything anyone said. One day he came home and began accusing me (as he usually did) of whatever it was that he had been told. He would never ask me about the situation. He would just make accusations. This time he became so violent that he tried to hurt me. My mom told me to run to my room and lock the door. He went up to my room and proceeded to knock the door down.

My mom told me to run so I packed a small duffle bag, with just under garments, jumped out my balcony window and ran for my life. I was so scared. I lived on the streets for ten days. I had no money for food. Finally, I found a quarter. I remember being so excited, but I had to make a decision. Do I eat or call for help? I decided that if I used the quarter to make a phone call, I would get food, drink, and shelter. I called my cousin, and she sent a cab for me. I stayed with her for a couple of days. While I was there, she had me call my mom.

My mom was so happy to hear my voice. She told me to come back home. I didn't want to go back but she had such sternness in her voice that I knew I had too. She spoke to my cousin, who took me back to my house. I was terrified but knew I had to obey. My dad gave my mom and me the silent treatment for what seemed like a month.

When I turned eighteen, I thought to myself "No one is going to tell me what to do anymore!" Rebellion became my new attitude. I began seducing Tony. I was tired of being called names and tired of the accusations. I wanted to be grown (an adult), and to me, that meant I should be having sex.

Because I loved Tony so much and we had a history between us, I thought, "Who better to have my first sexual experience with?" I started giving my parents a difficult time. They tried being harder on me, but I would lie to get my way, which made my life hell. Well, I showed them! I had sex......and sex with the boy I loved was the most wonderful experience.

Both of my parents did not have a relationship with Jesus Christ, neither did Tony nor myself. We both were acting, planning and doing everything against God's plans for our lives, and I got pregnant. What a shock! I remember thinking, "Oh my gosh!" What do we do now?" We were TERRIFIED! "Who do we speak to? Where do we turn?"

A year prior to this our dads had gotten into a boxing match that left a sour taste between both families. So we now found ourselves with nowhere to go; no one to speak to. We were so scared. We clung to each other and cried. We didn't know what to do.

"Abortion, yes abortion, that's what we'll do," is what we decided. With nowhere to go and no one to speak to that seemed to be our best option. I didn't want to have the abortion at all. Tony on the other hand thought, "well maybe that's the best thing" since he was not only scared, but realized it would be the easy way out since having a baby would trap him and change his life.

A week later at eight weeks pregnant, we went for the abortion. I cried and was sick to my stomach. I was told it was the size of a blood clot. I had passed plenty of blood clots. I knew exactly what they were but that didn't ease or change the pain in my heart. I remember turning around to look at Tony hoping he would say "Let's get out of here," or "Don't do it," ..... anything, but he didn't. I turned back around and went through the door. I never forgot that horrible feeling. I walked down a corridor and was told to put on a gown. The doctor and nurses entered the room and my nightmare began.

The smell of the room and the sounds of the machines haunted me. I was physically destroyed. I went home and laid in bed -- in the dark --- for two days, and cried. My uncle had died of cancer so my Mom and Grandma left for California. My Dad stayed home with us. He knew my periods were bad, so with my Mom and Grandma gone, it was easy for me to just stay in bed for two days and tell him it was a bad period.

Eventually, I had to get up and go to school and work. By the time my Mom returned home, I was able to disguise the emotions I felt from the loss of my baby as mourning for the loss of my uncle.

Tony and I continued dating. All I wanted to do was cry and talk about the abortion and my baby, our baby. Being a man ---- and a young one at that --- he was over it, but I couldn't get to that point. Soon it strained our relationship and we broke up. Because we loved each other, we had an on again, off again relationship. I wanted to be with him but I hated him. I just couldn't understand why I felt that way.

A year later we were engaged. I felt he owed me that since I gave him my virginity and aborted his baby, and I loved him. Four years later we married. There was total chaos. There were many arguments, drinking and partying. He worked late hours. He was rarely home and there were affairs. I cried and was miserable, but my love for him held strong.

I had two miscarriages in the mist of the chaos. I was miserable, but I would put on my happy face around everyone and anyone. I later learned it's what we do. Then we had our first son and I fell in love. I thanked God over and over again. Three years and eight months later we had a second son --- another joy and gift from God. I thanked God over and over again.

"Did God forgive me for killing my baby?" I wondered, but didn't know for sure. He did give me two sons….. but He didn't give me a girl, a daughter. He knew I wanted a daughter. Maybe that was part of my punishment. No daughter, a miserable marriage and a miserable life (except for our sons).

After eight years of marriage and two sons, I couldn't handle the pressures of life. I carefully planned one day and waited for Tony to leave for work. When the boys laid down for a nap I took out the gun we had. I was going to end my misery. I was going to take the lives of our sons' and then my own. That would solve all the pain and our boys wouldn't be a burden to anyone. Their Dad could continue living his life with no strings attached.

I grabbed the gun. I went in and out of the boys' room. I cried out to God…"Please God give me the strength to do this." Yes, I had the nerve to ask a loving God to give me the strength to commit murder again. I kept roaming back and forth. Suddenly the house phone rang. There was no Caller I.D. back then. I answered thinking it would be my mother. I didn't want her to worry. I wanted my husband to find us because I was so angry and bitter towards him. I hated him because of what he was putting me through.

It was a long time friend. She knew me so well. I was trying to control my voice and keep my throat from trembling. I had been crying intensely. I broke down and opened my heart to her. I didn't know she had accepted Jesus Christ as her Lord and Savior. (I didn't even know what that meant). My friend talked with me for a while and prayed. She then asked me to get a Bible. I refused. I just wanted to hang up and proceed with my plan. She persisted. I got the Bible. She asked me to read Romans 10:8-9. I did. She asked, "Do you know what that means?" I said, "No."

She asked if I believed Jesus Christ died for my sins and God raised Him up three days later. I said, "Yes, yes".Then I prayed to and asked Jesus into my heart. She barely heard me. I was drowning in tears. She asked again, and I answered her again. She then explained I had just accepted Jesus Christ as my Lord and Savior. My mind and emotions were being transformed. I was sobbing uncontrollably. She explained that I would be committing murder in the presence of Jesus Christ, God and the Holy Spirit, that had just been activated in my heart, soul and life. I slid down to the ground with the phone in my hand sobbing. God saved me and my children.

So here I am today to share my testimony. Life has been difficult but I've learned that with God ALL things are possible. During my transition and growth in the Word of God, I became disabled. I slowly learned I was God-abled. As I healed from my health issues and spiritually, through the Word of God I began to see more clearly.

I attended church one Saturday night. In the flyer was an invitation to volunteer at the Pregnancy Center. I read it and put it away. The following Monday the Holy Spirit placed it in my heart to call the Center, but I felt unworthy. Again the feeling came over me to call, but I felt useless. The third time was a very strong feeling so I called. An answering machine answered. I left a message looking up to the sky, saying out loud, "See God? No one answered." I took a shower, and when I got out, the phone rang. It was the Pregnancy Center.

I went for an interview on Thursday. As if she could see through me, the Director asked me, "Have you ever had an abortion?" I almost died! I broke down and sobbed, "Yes!"

I began my training and attended the Post Abortion Support Group. As difficult as it was to attend the group, I continued. I'm so blessed that I did. I hadn't realized that the abortion was like a cancer that had spread through ALL aspects of my life.

For the first time in my life, I've been able to see my life through God's eyes and not my own. I can finally breathe and live. Because of God's truth I've found my purpose in life. I now volunteer at the Pregnancy Center and enjoy every minute of it!

Janet's Journey of Healing
Jesus Our Redeemer

*I*t was 1988. I was 30, divorced, a mom to two children and pregnant. I didn't want to be pregnant for a lot of different reasons. I wasn't married. I didn't want a baby now --- and I didn't want my family and friends to know that I was having sex outside marriage --- so I made the decision to abort the life that was growing inside of me. After the procedure was finished, I stuffed down all the emotions and thoughts that were trying to make their way to the surface and continued with plans for my life. I resolved to be good for the rest of my life and hoped that would cancel out the abortion.

In 1992 I married Mike. He had custody of his two children and I had custody of my two. In 1994 we had another daughter, Elizabeth, and in 1996 our son, Ben, came along. We were the perfect family who lived in the comfortable two-story home in the suburbs. People said that we were like the Brady Bunch with three boys and three girls! I had everything I wanted. Why couldn't I quit thinking about the abortion? Why was I so unhappy? After all, when I scheduled the abortion, the woman told me that it was the best thing to do in my situation. It was legal. So what was my problem?

The problem was I had sinned against God and I knew it. What I didn't know was how to make it right. I grew more and more depressed. I was dying inside but I continued to keep the abortion a secret from everyone and kept trying to fix it by myself. After attempts at counseling and antidepressants I finally surrendered the secret to Jesus --- 12 years later --- on November 4, 2000. I told Him how sorry I was and asked Him to help me. As I look back and think about that night I am so amazed at how well He knew how to approach me. First of all, it was just Him and me – no one else came in the room the whole time --- second, He let me talk it all the way through and express all the emotions that had been bottled up inside for so long; third, He gave me what I wanted and so desperately needed, His unconditional love and acceptance.

He didn't just save me from eternal separation from God.....He redeemed me! He bought my freedom with His blood! For twelve years I had kept that awful secret and just like that ---- in one night --- I was free from it! I fell head over heels in love with Jesus because He rescued me from the pit of hopelessness.

Even though He forgave me and set me free from the fear of death and punishment that night, my journey to healing had just started. I needed to acknowledge the loss of my child and give him a name. I chose to call him David because King David was a man who knew about being redeemed by God's love.

I can't hold him now, but I will hold him in Heaven. It was painful to allow myself to feel the emotions of grief but it was necessary to move forward. I learned the importance of God's Word and how it changes our heart and minds to be like Jesus. Now I help women experience His love and redemption by sharing His Word and my story of healing with them.

Psalm 103:3-5 says He forgives all our sins and heals us completely – physically, emotionally, and spiritually. He redeems us from death and instead crowns us with love and tender mercies. He fills our life with good things. These words are true. They were true for King David when he wrote them. They were true for me on November 4, 2000, and they are true for you today. Thankfully, this story doesn't end with my healing. He asked me to reach out to others who are hurting from the pain of abortion. This is the beauty God gave me for the ashes of my sin. Instead of guarding my secret, I share it with others to give them hope. Jesus can be trusted with the broken parts within us all. He is the only One who can truly heal our wounds. And after the healing is complete, He will use our stories to help others.

In the spring of 2001 I secretly prayed the prayer of Isaiah, "Lord here I am send me." Then I forgot about it. Also in the spring of 2001 my husband, Mike, gave his life to the Lord. Since then our lives have been turned upside down and inside out!

When I became a new creation in Christ I would get up early and sit quietly reading the Bible. It didn't always make sense but it always moved me – either to tears or to joy or to action. God was gracious and connected us with wonderful Christian friends. We were like sponges soaking up all we could from His Word and from the body of Christ. We soon stepped out in faith and began tithing (at 5% - we were too afraid to do the full 10% at that time). I spent a lot of time talking with God during my early morning quiet times. (Working 40 hours a week and caring for 6 kids didn't leave a lot of time for quiet!)

It was during one of these early morning conversations in 2002 when I was asking God what to do about our financial situation. I felt like He said "just put up a 'For Sale By Owner' sign in front of the house". I shared this with my husband and he thought it sounded like a good idea but it was a full 6 months before we acted on it.

The same day we put up the sign, a couple in our neighborhood stopped by and they bought our house! They had a small house around the corner so we moved in and rented from them. A couple of months later my husband took an early retirement package and all of a sudden we were completely out of debt with money in the bank. We liked how all of that worked! We became more confident in following God's Word and began tithing 10%. Our plan was for me to continue working at my full-time job while Mike built up his business and then we were going to move to Florida. In the spring of 2003 I was having another conversation with the Lord and it went like this:

Me: "Father we can't move to Florida yet because I work at Lilly and that is our financial security until Mike's business is solid."

Father: "Lilly is not your financial security, I AM!"

So, I shared the conversation with my husband and he said, "OK, let's move to Florida!" This time I was a little scared but I gave my notice at work. A co-worker of mine told me about a good company in Florida she used to work for and gave me a contact name. I emailed them and got a job interview. I had an unused airline ticket to Florida so I flew to Orlando for the interview. They hired me. By July of 2003 we had moved into a new house in Clermont, Florida. Wow!!

Remember my Isaiah prayer, "Lord send me?" Well, in November of 2006 while riding to the beach with my family, I was reading Isaiah 61 and the words began to sound like a job description to me. I felt in my heart that God was sending me to minister to women who had abortions. He said to create a safe place for those hurt by abortion to come for healing and restoration. I had a lot of work to do. I didn't know anything about abortion.

I love the wisdom of the Lord. The first thing He did was connect me to people who did. I met June Barrow with Southport Presbyterian Church, Christine Land, Mary Comm with In Our Midst, Synda Masse with Ramah International, Lori Wren with Reveille Ministries, Sandy Epperson, Carmem Carmo & Myrtzie Levell with First Life Pregnancy Center and Mary Lou Hendry with the Florida Baptist Children's Home. This list is so extensive I will apologize now for those I forget to mention.

Everyone I spoke with told me the same thing….. you need to go through a healing Bible Study that deals with abortion. I found a pregnancy center in Orlando called First Life that offered post abortion healing. That's where I met Sandy Epperson who was the Director of the center at that time and Myrtzie Levell who was heading up the HOPE program.

I met with Sandy in January of 2007 and shared with her what God was asking me to do. She agreed to take me through their post abortion healing Bible Study called First Steps. Upon completion of the Study, they held a memorial service for our babies. My husband and children attended the service with me. David's life was no longer a secret.

The next step in my training was to co-lead a post abortive Bible study. I was very nervous about it, but Myrtzie served as leader. She was so full of mercy that it was easy to lead alongside her. It was during the First Steps Bible Study that I met Cindy Fitzgibbon. God connected our hearts right away and I am privileged to call her my sister in Christ. I was very comfortable serving at First Life and longed to continue working with Sandy & Myrtzie, but God was very clear that He wanted me to serve in the community where I lived.

That was really scary but God, in His perfect wisdom, sent Cindy and me out together. For the next year Cindy and I ministered to post abortive women together. It was such a blessing to see the women receive freedom and peace. Cindy and I both felt so privileged to be a part of such a wonderful ministry of the Lord! Cindy and Myrtzie continue to work with post abortive women at First Life in Orlando. They are awesome women of God ---full of grace and His love.

One day I went with Cindy to a local abortion facility and prayed outside. It was a bittersweet experience, difficult, yet filled with hidden blessings from the Lord. I built an altar to the Lord that day because I had returned to a familiar place with a changed heart. Lamentations 3:22-24 says:

"Through the Lord's mercies we are not consumed, because His compassions fail not, they are new every morning. Great is Your

faithfulness. The Lord is my portion, says my soul, therefore, I hope in Him."

After being at an abortion facility and seeing the devastating impact abortion has on individuals, families and our nation, I knew it was time to expand the ministry to a full service pregnancy center. God was giving me a passion for the pregnancy center ministry. Using the First Life Center in Orlando as our model we opened Beauty for Ashes Center in February of 2011. The struggles have been tremendous and many times I have wanted to quit, but God promises to finish the good work He starts within us; and for that I am forever grateful.

So this is what I have learned on my journey…..

The love of God is like a refreshing wave that sweeps us off our feet. Sometimes His love can be frightening because we don't know where it will lead us. But if we allow His love to overtake our hearts, He will sweep us off our feet and take us to the mountaintop. When we believe that He is always with us and His outstretched hands are always there to help us up after a fall, we will keep coming back for more of His love. Isn't that what every little girl dreams of – a dashing Prince Charming to sweep her off her feet and lead her on a life of adventure while making sure no harm comes to her?

Take it from a formerly fearful woman who has been transformed into Daddy's little girl…He can be trusted with your heart! Today I live for Him instead of for myself. Today I am filled with hope and the love of Jesus. It is a good life; better than I ever dreamed!

Kaye's Journey of Healing
Depending on God

I am writing this to tell you of the worse and best decision of my life. I'm a 35 year old wife and mother of three children. I have a college education and live in a middle class neighborhood. I'm a believer in Christ, faithful church member, and Sunday school teacher. That is where it all ended for me. I did all things thinking that I had a relationship with God and I knew who He was. I did not. Here is my story of the worst and best decision of my life.

One early morning, I bought a pregnancy test because I noticed that I missed my cycle. But then again, I also had an IUD so it was common for me to miss a cycle here and there.

I woke up that morning, went into the bathroom and took a test. It was positive. I ran into the room where my husband was and told him to wake up. I told him the test was positive. He looked in disbelief and said nothing. I was crying. I did not want this baby. I was at a point in my life where I was getting me back.

I had plans to finish my degree. I was losing weight. My marriage was in a solid place. NOW THIS LORD?! No way could I have this child. NO WAY! Right then and there I decided to abort my baby. I called around to make an appointment and scheduled it for a week later --- Saturday, January 21, 2011.

That whole week I did not talk to my husband. He did not talk to me. I was in a daze. That whole week all I could think about was getting rid of it before it was too late. I did not pray or go to church that week. I knew what I was about to do was wrong but I made up mind to do it…and that was that.

Then the night before the abortion, my husband woke me up and said, "Are you ready to deal with the blood on your hands for this death?"

At first I was really irritated because he hadn't spoken to me the entire week. Not once did he say, "Baby, it will be fine. I will stick with you…I will be with you." Nothing! Nothing at all --- except was I ready to have blood on my hands. I didn't respond. Instead I turned over and went to sleep.

The next day I woke up, got dressed and left. Once again, he never got up to stop me. From that point on, I was sure that my husband didn't want the baby either. I drove to the place. At first I was nervous because I knew deep down inside I should not do this.

I was so determined to go through with it because I wanted the life I had and not the life with a new baby. Just plain selfish. All that morning, all I heard once I got in the place was that it was a simple, safe procedure. The only thing I would have to deal with was the mental part of it.

While waiting my turn, all I heard from the pastor on the street was that I will have this blood on my hands. In my mind, I couldn't hear anything but hate coming over the mega phone. But I was determined to get rid of the baby. Finally my turn came. I walked down the hall to the room. The nurse told me to undress from the waist down. I did. At that point, I had second thoughts, but went through with it anyway. The doctor came in to turn on the machine, I turned my head to the side and told my baby bye. I cried one tear and it was over. So I thought…

The best decision of my life started two days later after the abortion. I woke up crying my eyes out. I couldn't sleep all that night. I wanted to end my life. I wanted nothing to do with my husband or kids. I saw myself as this awful person. I wanted God to end my life.

For what I did, I deserved death. I felt so dirty and unclean. I didn't have an appetite anymore. I was a mess. Every day, I wanted my life to end. I wanted the pain to stop. I kept asking myself over and over again how I could have done this. This baby was conceived in love.

My husband didn't know what to do with me. My children kept asking me why was I so sad all the time. My life was a mess. I had to do something. That Tuesday I went through the phone book and called the Pregnancy Center. I was in need of someone to talk to who could tell me what to do with all of these emotions. I called to set up an appointment and was told to come in today. I ran to the Center and couldn't get the door open fast enough before I was greeted by my counselor. She took me into the client room and I cried my heart out. I was talking and crying about what I did and how I felt.

She was listening and rubbing my back. She made me feel calm. For the first time in two weeks since this had happened, I felt peace. I don't know if she was praying for me as I was talking, but I felt peace right there in that room with her. When I was done, she began to tell me her story.

She made me feel calm. She shared her life story and we realized that we had similar stories. She made me look at my situation for the sin it was. But also, that I was forgiven by God because of His Son, Jesus. She told me that God knew I would do this before the beginning of time and had me come to them for my healing.

Now I told you in the beginning I had been a believer, so I knew what she told me was true. The one thing that was different now is that I truly received the Lord in my heart.

After that meeting, I had a very long and hard recovery ahead of me. That year I sought out the Lord every day. I read my Bible daily. This gave me strength through my midnight panic attacks, self-doubts, and kept me going... one step at a time. My husband and I became stronger in the Lord and together went to counseling at First Steps Post Abortion Recovery class at the Pregnancy Center.

The First Steps class was nothing like I expected. My husband and I went to the first class and were nervous. I thought I would be judged for what I did. But when we arrived, we were welcomed with open arms. The mentors were very understanding. Each week, they showed us step-by-step how to get through the grieving process of what we did and how we were forgiven for our sin. The mentors used Biblical scriptures and their own personal testimonies. This process helped us to understand all the emotions we were going through at the time. We were able to cry and express ourselves openly with the class.

With every homework assignment we were seeing God's healing at work in us. He showed us His power of forgiveness and redemption. We never thought the class would have helped us so much but it did. Had we not taken this class, we would have never healed from the abortion.

Later that year, I was asked by my counselor to become a mentor at the center. At first, I was thinking I wasn't ready yet. I was not qualified to teach or mentor anyone. Who was I to talk to about the Lord when I didn't seek Him before my abortion?

I had a lot of emotions I was going through. I agreed to sit in on the class and help out in the background. But as time went on, I sat there and began to realize the Lord could and would use me. Satan wanted me to take my sin and be ashamed and hide forever. God on the other hand, wanted to use what I went through to help others. After they are the healed, then He will be glorified. So I became a mentor for the fall classes.

I told you this abortion was the worst and best decision of my life. The worst decision of my life because I killed my baby for selfish reasons and didn't give him the opportunity to live. This is a decision I will have to live with for the rest of my life.

It is the best decision because I'm developing a closer relationship with the Lord, and He is using me and my sin to help others who went through or are going through the same situation. It made me totally depend on the Lord for everything and able to recognize Satan's attacks in my life. Also, I now know God's unconditional love for me.

To God be the Glory,
Kaye

Patricia's Journey of Healing
I Am a New Creation

My name is Patricia and my desire is you will be able to identify with my story and understand that you are not alone, and your story is just as important to God as my story. My prayer is for you to find the strength to take he first step toward your journey of healing.

I must start by saying at the age of eighteen, my life was already broken into pieces. I was born into a dysfunctional home where alcohol was very important to my father. My mother was not a loving or an affectionate woman because she was full of pain and bitterness she could not let go.

My father decided to abandon his family and I suffered the aftermath of abandonment at the early age of five. Because of my experience with having a father who abandoned me and an unloving mother, I grew up to be a very insecure, unhealthy young woman with low self-esteem. Subsequently I found myself in situations of abuse and violence over and over again.

I was looking for help, love and protection from someone in a world that I didn't understand. Because I was so naïve, I started to look for a man to love me. All I wanted was to be loved.

I did have a boyfriend and for me that was very important because I needed to feel loved. It seemed like I had everything going for me...for a moment. I had a boyfriend and a great future as a singer. I was in the most prestigious folk dance company in my country. I felt like everything was fine. My life seemed perfect until I found out that I was several months pregnant --- and what was most alarming --- I found out I was pregnant with twins! Oh, gosh! What should I do?

I was feeling confused. I was full of fear and feeling empty. I felt so alone. It was extremely painful with all the different emotions that I was feeling. My perfect world had collapsed all around me. It made me feel like I was that little five year old girl again, abandoned by her father, but now with an adult mind and body and a big problem to solve.

I made my way to the car where my older sister was waiting for me. I felt like I was going to pass out. Literally, at any time I could faint. As I went into the car, I did not say anything. The pain in my face said it all.

For a few seconds it was completely silent. Then the silence was interrupted by the voice of my sister who was upset, but sad at the same time. She was giving me all the possible reasons why I should end my pregnancy. She let me know that she knew of a place where I could get an abortion and said her husband would help with expenses. We would tell our mother I would spend the weekend with them. In my weakness I agreed with her plan.

I remember sitting in the waiting room of the doctor's office with many people. No thoughts were going through my mind. I felt numb. I felt empty of emotion….until the nurse startled me by calling my name. I jumped, and then she led me to the office where the doctor was.

He immediately began to explain the whole process and the amount of time it would take. After this, he left me with the nurse, who gave me two pills and showed me where I could change my clothes and put on a hospital gown. A terrible cold started to take over my body. Again, I began feeling like I would faint any minute, but then the nurse's voice made me react and all of my body started shaking.

I went out to lie on the operating table. Then the doctor started the abortion. It was so painful. I was feeling like my entire life was being changed. My life was stripped away forever. The abortion not only stripped my two babies' lives away, it did mine as well. It made me feel so empty inside. The nurse assured me everything would be fine.

NO. That was not true. Nothing was right! Something in me was dying besides my two babies...besides me. All I wanted at that moment was to finish right then. I wanted to run away from that place and for the pain to end. I wanted to move forward with my life and put this nightmare in the deepest part of my heart, and not look back and never have to go there again.

Finally! Those minutes that seemed timeless had ended. Suddenly, I was in a recovery room. I felt a big void, but I was trying to convince myself I could move on with my life and the career I loved. And that is exactly what happened. Everything was fine for a while; travel, successes, not having to spend much time at home, new friendships, new relationships. I began consuming more alcohol, using it as a measure of escape from the sadness, fear and pain that was in my heart and soul.

A second pregnancy happened, and then a third. They took me by surprise. I had buried and forgotten the deep pain that was caused by my first abortion, so it was not a difficult decision to have another abortion --- knowing that the father of the babies did not want anything to do with them, and that abortion was his one condition for moving forward with our relationship.

All the same fear and pain I experienced the first time, re-occurred and my mind was locked. In my shame and brokenness, it seemed I was always going by myself to the clinic as the broken little five year old girl having to make these big decisions alone. Each time I would leave the abortion clinic I would feel empty and sick. I would have a thousand questions going through my head. I had to force myself to put one foot in front of the other, and sometimes I seriously considered the possibility of suicide to end the pain, loneliness, and shame.

The years passed almost in the same way. The biggest difference was that I was drinking alcohol all the time. Around the age of 25, I realized that I had been pregnant for four months. As always, my first thought was "abort!" So I asked for help from a friend to help me go to the hospital to discuss costs. I clearly remember the cold and fear seizing over me that day ----and even more so when I listened to the person who was going to perform the abortion. He told me that he could do it but with the condition that I sign a paper that stated I was 100% responsible if something happened. Because my pregnancy was advanced, I could die on the table.

Total silence. I left that place feeling empty and sat on the edge of the street crying inconsolably. I tried to explain to my friend what the doctor had said. The only thing my friend could say was, "What did I want to do?"

I didn't know. I just knew that my mother and my brothers couldn't find out. We sat in silence for a few minutes until I could stop crying and have the courage to return home. On the way back --- with a thousand thoughts going through my head --- I decided that the best I could do was to move out of my mother's house, and try talking to the baby's father with whom I did not have a good relationship anymore.

So I did. I went to the house of one of the owners of the place where I was working at that time, with just a small suitcase and no money. After that, I called the baby's father for help. He assured me that the baby was not his, but decided to help me and wait for the baby to be born to find out.

The days passed and I was feeling so alone and abandoned in the house where I had taken refuge. I knew I couldn't stay any longer, so I found the courage to call my sister and tell her what

and gratitude, I attended each class. I fully opened my heart to every word the leader said and the other women who shared their stories. I let God in His infinite love and tenderness continue doing His work in me.

It was a wonderful journey. Sometimes it was painful, but each time God came with His word and healed all my wounds. Little by little, I understood grace, forgiveness, and mercy of God because I needed to be freed from the bondage I was in. The guilt and shame kept me from moving forward for many years.

By completing this Bible Study, I enjoy total freedom and experience a desire to help other women who have gone through the painful process of abortion find faith and hope. I can also live fully with the Word that God impressed upon my heart.

"Therefore if any man be in Christ, he is a new creature; old things are passed away; behold all things become new."

~ 2 Corinthians 5:17

Christy's Journey of Healing
Behind the Smile

My story begins at age 16 when I was attending a prayer meeting for my boyfriend's brother who had been killed in a tragic car accident. One of the local churches invited the youth of our community in to help us process his death and pray.

Jesus was tugging on my heart so I stepped forward to begin my journey with Him. It wasn't until years later the next significant steps on this journey would be walked out. Following that prayer meeting, I had essentially moved away from Him, not fully knowing how to develop a relationship with Him. Later, He found me in a deep, dark pit where He reached down to offer His loving hand to help lift me out into forgiveness, healing and freedom.

After High School graduation, I began to make plans to attend college in the fall. With excitement for what my future held, I celebrated my accomplishment with my family and boyfriend during a summer vacation at the beach. It was there that my boyfriend and I decided we were ready to have sex. The result: an unplanned pregnancy. I was 18. I felt like a child myself and now had to make a choice about what would be done about that child.

I was devastated and in shock. I was so heartbroken. I couldn't fathom how in the world I would make this decision and that someday this would be in the past! I told my older sister, and then with gut wrenching pain and many tears shed, I eventually shared with my parents. My father silently supported me while my mother lovingly said: "I will support whatever decision you make," believing it was mine to determine.

Even with support, this felt so heavy. I felt so alone, so confused and so desperate. After learning the news, my boyfriend wanted to get married, but I was leaning toward adoption, not feeling equipped to raise a child and certain we did not need to be married at the time.

"What about my future? How can I raise this child? What about college? What will people in our small (gossip-filled) town think of me? What will my grandparents think? They will be so disappointed in me." My thoughts and fears consumed me! I prayed to ask God to forgive me for the decision I was going to make and to take the baby's soul, keep him and take care of him. In my spirit, I questioned: was this enough?

During this time, much of society believed that a fetus was only a blob of tissue and a woman had the right to choose what would happen to her body when she faced an unwanted pregnancy. I bought into this, believing I could make this "problem" go away with a simple choice, based on the counseling I received at the clinic. This of course was a lie. I exchanged one so-called "problem" for a far greater one!

I will never forget entering the full waiting room, looking around at the other girls who waited to be taken back for their procedures, and feeling so strangely alone. Our eyes never met, as we all tried desperately to mentally escape this reality.

I lay on the table at the clinic and had my child removed from my body. Not only was my child's life taken but so was my own. I became emotionally numb. No attempt to distract myself from the cold reality of where I was and what I was truly doing comforted my soul. My mom drove me away from this cold place.

I remember leaving the clinic, staring blankly out the window with raindrops falling down the car window --- a symbolic picture of the years which would follow. Nineteen years of shame, pain, depression, self-condemnation and judgment all became my emotional prison and my dark, ugly pit.

Many times my aborted child would come to my mind and heart over the years. I'd ask myself, "How old would he be now? Or what would he look like? Or what does God think about what I did? What does He think about me?!" Usually the condemning reply to myself would be: How dare you?! "How could God possibly love you after the horrible thing you did?!"

One sleepless night after waking from a dream related to my abortion, I went to the internet searching the words abortion and depression. I came close to answering God's wooing me to Him for healing as I was connected to an online Bible study.

A tender-hearted counselor/mentor, who had walked the same path reached out to me and encouraged me to sign up for their study along with one-on-one counseling with her. I was not ready to face my pain and continued to keep my mask on with my pain hiding just behind the smile I put on my face.

With the pregnancy of each of my sons, I struggled to cope with the shame and loss surrounding my abortion. My soul and heart were wounded; pregnancy brought me deeply face to face with this reality. I believed God had every right to take the child I was carrying for what I had done, as a way to atone for my horrible sin. These babies were babies I wanted, I longed for, ones I had planned for yet would He punish me in this way for what I had done? Uncertain, I clung to them tightly holding my breath with thoughts of the possibility that He could take them at any moment.

When my sons were toddlers, I decided they deserved to have a loving relationship with God even though I did not. I began to search for a church home. Little did I know He was directing my journey straight into His loving arms through the love of my children. I began to get connected, serving in ministry and growing in my daily journey with Him, yet there was still a huge wall between Him and me. Reading through the list of Bible studies my church was offering, I casually overlooked the post-abortion healing study only to opt for a Beth Moore study thinking: "eh, I'm okay with all that."

It wasn't until I witnessed an amazing woman sharing the testimony of her two abortions, before the entire congregation, that I felt God powerfully yanking at my heart! She stood onstage with her head held up, her eyes looking into ours as she claimed to be an oak of righteousness, a planting of the Lord, for His glory! I was amazed and moved to tears. Everyone was.

She was leading a study which offered healing and forgiveness. My heart leapt within my chest crying out: GO FORWARD! SIGN UP! This beautiful woman of God later shared with me how shocked she was when I quickly ran up to her after the service to sign my name on the list. At that time, I didn't care who saw me, what they thought or how painful it might prove to be. I was so ready to receive His healing and tear down the wall that kept me from being exactly who He created me to be! I no longer wanted to live in the prison, the awful, ugly, dark pit with my broken heart in pieces.

Completing the study, I received healing but not without challenges or facing my deeply seated pain. Out of the pit, I felt His love, forgiveness, restoration, joy and amazingly, song and color took on new life! After completing the study, I was baptized by my leader just before Christmas as my family, including my parents, watched me rise up out of the water a new creation. The other side of healing felt amazing. Such a heavy burden had been lifted. The wall was removed!

A few years later God took me even further along the journey as He molded me for leadership. Now, I stand before others, the oak of righteousness, the planting of the Lord, for His Glory! With the honor of witnessing other women finding their healing journey, I have been facilitating study groups off and on for 10 years.

Only boasting in His power, He has enabled me to travel to China in honor of my lost child, to take the post-abortion materials to two shelters where girls who have been removed from sex trafficking live and learn how to walk in Christ's freedom.

In 2012, I entered a graduate program to train even further. I'm now on my way toward becoming a licensed mental health counselor. Passionately, I am called to share with others how to find their journey toward living a full abundant life. Never in a million years would I have guessed my Heavenly Father would not only heal my ugliest, darkest most painful sin but He would use that same sin to make me an instrument in other's healing journey. I am blessed to be a part of this mission. The journey continues.

Behind the Smile

Cold and dark, this pit of mine, I put myself here.
Just as well if I stay, I don't even feel alive.
I wear a smile but look in my eyes, can't you see the pain?
See me, see me, somebody see me, help me live again.
Help me now my heart is broken, God, my God,
Don't you see?!
My silent cry is deafening. Don't you hear the pain
Behind the smile?

The "other side" sounds real nice but can it really be?
"Trust me," you say, say to me, I will set you free!
…Free to fly
…Free to dance
…Free to sing again.
…Free to live
…Free to love
Love....even myself?

Look in the mirror, something's new, can't really
say just what.
In my eyes a beautiful light, put there by His love.
And in my heart there's laughter and song,
there's color to my soul.
You see me smile; ask me why, I don't mind telling it all.
Peel the layers off for you, so you can see,
 the love behind the smile.

Janete's Journey of Healing
His Promises

I was born and raised by my Christian mother, but when I was about 16 years old I started to question the church and everything that had to do with it. From that point on I was focused on ME only, my career, my friends, and my life.

At 18 I went to college and a whole different world opened to me. new friends, new home, new life. My high school sweetheart started to look less appealing when I met the coolest guy on campus. The only problem was I wasn't cool enough for him.

I started to try to impress him and my peers. I broke up with my boyfriend, and started to go out with different guys. On my school break, at 23 I got pregnant, with someone I barely knew or wanted to know. I was scared of my family, and I knew that a baby could ruin my plans for graduation, career and my life.

It was my last year in college. I had too much to live for. I decided to have an abortion, and a friend helped me find a good place. I didn't know anything about abortion. I actually was against it, and it was illegal in my country. I don't remember the details but I remember walking in and talking to a doctor about the procedure. What he painted for me was the simplest, easiest, best solution for my problem. From there I was directed to a room where the nurse put me to sleep. Then I remember waking up in another room where my friend was waiting for me.

The sense of relief didn't last long. Thoughts about the baby and the decision had to be erased from my mind. I started to look for something to fulfill that emptiness in my heart... drinking, partying and new people.

After I graduated from college, the reality started to sink in. I met another guy and we kind of lived together, until I found out that he had other women. I broke up with him and 2 weeks later found out I was pregnant again. I panicked. He gave me no other option, so I agreed. I went back to the same clinic, with him; the same doctor, the same room. This time I woke up to an anxious ex-boyfriend that couldn't wait to drop me off and get rid of me.

He left me alone. This time it was harder. I cried for hours and decided that nobody would ever make me feel that way again. I would start new again and forget about everything, focus on my career and my future. I never thought the abortions would have such a negative impact on my life, my relationships and me.

For twenty seven years, I tried everything the world had to offer. I did all the wrong things I could do --- partying, bad relationships, abortions, drinking, smoking --- but nothing could fill my heart. I was always lonely, and looking for the next thing to make me happy.

After every party, achievement, graduation, I was alone and anxious for the next diversion; always empty and looking for someone or something that could make me feel better, accepted and complete.

My mom never stopped telling me I needed to go to church Even though I never told her about my abortions, out of fear and embarrassment, she knew something was wrong with me. My younger brother became a Christian. He tried to tell me about his new life, but I still wasn't ready to hear it. I thought I had gone too far. God was punishing me. He would never forgive me.

Even though I worked with three Christian people in the ten years I lived here I was never invited to a church. My friends were not Christians. They accepted me and invited me to parties and on trips.

I never totally forgot my Christian foundation. It's what kept me out of a lot of trouble. Also I started to feel the need to find a church. My mom always asked me if I was going to church, and I always gave her a good reason why I was not.

At forty three years old, I finally decided to find a church. I invited my boyfriend at the time to go with me, since I didn't have the courage to go alone. We went to a small church by my house and I instantly felt the peace. I cried but it felt like going back home.

Three months later we were both baptized, and since then my life began to slowly change. I started to see the kind of relationship we had and all the problems he had, with no signs of change. We broke up, and a friend suggested another church to me.

I wanted to be close to the Lord; to serve him. I wanted to volunteer at my church. I found the Pregnancy Center, and my journey to healing started. When I thought I would be helping, I actually realized I needed help. I just didn't know it. It wasn't easy and many times I thought I wasn't good enough and my sins were too big to be forgiven. Thanks to God's grace and mercy, He put the right people and His plan into my life so I could learn about His Love. I forgave myself; I learned to be thankful for His love, grace and mercy for sinners like me. I learned I could use my experience to witness to others.

I stopped listening to the enemy's lies and started listening to Jesus. I accepted what He had done for me at the Cross, and let Him transform my heart. I accepted the work of the Holy Spirit, and I thank God for His love, mercy, grace and forgiveness.

Being a disciple of Jesus Christ is the most important decision I made in my life. Although I'm still struggling and learning to "sanctify" my life, I know how far I have walked. I don't want to go back. I feel His peace. I have hope, and I'm stronger and content, even through life's storms.

My Lord and Savior didn't promise that life would be easier, but certainly it is worth it. His promises are for eternity. Now I just want to let the Holy Spirit work on my heart, and use me to fulfill God's purpose in my life. I will never walk alone again. All Glory be to our God!!!

Myrtzie's Journey of Healing
Walking With My Head Held High

Public School to Private School

After finishing the sixth grade in public school, my parents decided to send me to a private school. I found out it was very hard to fit in with a group of kids who had been together for seven years. Most of the kids at this school started out together in kindergarten. I left a school full of friends and ended up in a school where I had to start all over again.

The first year I was hard at work trying to fit in. I made some friends. Then I had a boy ask me to be his girlfriend. I said yes and we were a couple for about two months. Then I broke up with him, which made him very angry.

He began to spread rumors about me. He told all our peers as well as the teachers that I did drugs and was sexually active. He even told them I was bi-sexual. This didn't go over well in a private school. Even the faculty began to treat me differently.

Toward the end of the year I felt so alone. I begged my parents to take me out and let me go back to public school so I could be with the friends I had grown up with. But to no avail, I was sent back.

My eighth grade year was one of the most horrible experiences of my life. I had to go to school every day with my peers making fun of me. They all judged me and believed that I was this horrible person. I'll never forget one day in gym class. It was time to choose teams for a kickball game. They had picked teams and I was the last one standing to be picked. Then they argued about how neither team wanted me.

I heard all the belittling comments; my heart was breaking inside. Every day at school was a living nightmare. Then on Halloween night I met a boy from my neighborhood. He gave me some positive attention and I ate it up.

I needed him so much. I needed to feel loved and accepted, so when he told me he loved me I believed every word that he said. I would do anything for him, including sleep with him. This relationship became my hideaway from the hell I had to live in everyday at school. My relationship with this boy became the most important thing in my life. This boy was so important he was like my god.

He was my everything; I was so in love with him. I put him above everything. Then my parents found out that we were seeing each other and told me I couldn't see him because I was thirteen and he was three years older than I. I was in middle school and he was in high school.

Since my parents forbade us from seeing each other, we sneaked around. I didn't care if I got caught. He was the only thing or person that mattered to me. Then when I found out that he was dating other girls the entire time, I was heartbroken. I felt rejected again. I can remember feeling so alone. I had no friends and now no boyfriend.

I was devastated. I was so hurt. I felt like I was going to die. I cried so much it made my whole body hurt. I became so obsessed with him. I would walk by his house to see if I could see him or see if his car was there. I would call him just to hear his voice. It was like I was a heroin addict and he was my heroin.

I wanted him back so badly I was willing to try anything. I thought maybe if he saw me with another guy he would get jealous. Then maybe he would realize that he loved me and he would want me back. That idea backfired on me.

I started dating another guy and ended up getting pregnant. I told my best friend that I had missed my period so she took me to an abortion clinic to get a pregnancy test. As I waited for my test result to come in, it seemed like it was taking forever. I was so scared. My body was literally shaking. Then the lady came in and told me my test came out positive.

Instantly this wave of fear came over me. She asked me if I wanted to make an appointment for an abortion. I didn't even take time to think about it, because I knew if I thought about it I would change my mind. So I made the appointment for two weeks later. Afterwards I went home and called the boy and told him "I'm pregnant and I am getting an abortion and you are paying half." I didn't give him a chance to say yes or no.

Even though I had made up my mind to have the abortion, so many thoughts were going through my mind during the two weeks that followed. "How could I disappoint my parents any more than I already have?"

"What would my friends think of me?" "How could I be a good mother at the age of fifteen?"

I was so scared and it was such a paralyzing fear. But the fear won over and I decided to stick with my decision to have the abortion.

The Abortion

The birth father paid half and my best friend's cousin helped me get the rest of the money. I told my parents I was spending the night at my best friend's house for the weekend, so I was all set for my appointment.

My friend and her cousin brought me to the clinic. I remember sitting in the waiting room which was packed. There were even people waiting outside. I was so scared and I had so many thoughts going through my head. I had to keep talking myself through this. I had no other choice.

Finally, they called my name and brought me back to a little office where they explained what the procedure would be like and how long it would take. I was given two valiums and taken in the back to this room where they had me sit on a medical table with stirrups.

I had never been to a gynecologist before, so this was very scary to me. Then the abortionist started the procedure. It was so painful. I could see my stomach rippling and it felt like they were sucking my whole insides out. The nurse kept squeezing my hand assuring me that everything would be okay.

In my mind and heart I knew it wasn't going to be okay. My heart was screaming inside and I wanted them to stop, but it was too late --- too late for my baby and too late for me to go back and undo what was already done. The actual procedure took about ten to fifteen minutes, but it felt like forever.

Then they took me into the recovery room. This room had about ten recliner chairs in it. They made me sit for about fifteen minutes and checked on me to see if everything was okay. After about an hour or so they said I could go home.

I remember being relieved it was all over with, but at the same time I had such an empty feeling. All I could do was cry. We went home and I slept for the rest of the weekend. I couldn't talk much. Whenever I tried to talk I would just cry. After the weekend was over, I went home and tried to act like nothing happened.

The Aftermath

Later the next month I felt like I was going crazy. I kept wondering what would have happened if I didn't get that abortion. I would stay in my room not wanting to leave, I would stick a pillow under my shirt and look at myself in the mirror to see what I would have looked like if I were still pregnant. I had such an empty feeling. My heart would just ache.

One day I went to the grocery store and saw someone giving out free puppies. I saw this adorable tiny black and brown Dotson Beagle mix that I just had to have. I took the bow off that was tied around her neck because I was going to tell my parents that I found her.

When I got home I did just that. I told them that I found her. Later my mother talked to the Winn Dixie manager and he told her that there was someone out in front of the store giving out free puppies. Even though she found out, they still allowed me to keep her. I named her Princess.

Princess became the replacement of my baby I aborted. I treated her just like a baby. That seemed to help fill the emptiness for a short while. Still I tried to act like nothing had happened. I walked around with attitude; with a chip on my shoulder.

I tried very hard to keep myself together, but depression set in and I had to try something to make me feel better. I tried drinking. I tried drugs. I even tried more sex. Nothing worked. I thought I only had one choice left to stop the pain that I was feeling so deep in my heart. I decided to end my life.

I took a bottle of aspirin and went and lay on the couch waiting to die. My mom noticed my chest beating rapidly and she asked what was wrong with me. I told her nothing, but she kept insisting so I told her what I had done. She and my dad took me to the Emergency Room where they pumped my stomach. I remember that was the first time I saw my dad cry.

I was forced to see a counselor for a while, but I never told her about my abortion. I lied to her instead and told her I wanted to die because my boyfriend didn't love me anymore.

New Boyfriend

A year went by and I was still making a lot of bad choices. I still felt like I was dying inside and it was a challenge to make it through each day. Then one morning my best friend and I were meeting her cousin at Winn Dixie where he worked. He was there with his co-worker Tim whom he introduced me to. We hit it off right away.

I was telling him stupid jokes and he laughed at them anyway. He asked me for my phone number before we left for the beach. I was excited because he seemed like a real nice guy.

He waited three days before he called and asked me out on a date. I said yes and we started to date. This guy was different than all the other guys I had dated or been with. He would open the door for me and treated me with a lot of respect.

He got me to go back to church with him. We really liked each other; eventually we got close enough to talk about our past with each other. I decided to share with him my deep dark secret about having an abortion. I really thought that after he found out, he wouldn't want to be with me anymore.

But to my surprise he told me that he had a girlfriend in his past who had had an abortion. He mentioned that he wasn't too happy with her for doing that and said that he wished she hadn't had the abortion. In spite of my secret, he still accepted me and we continued to date.

Our relationship was really moving forward. We met each other's family and started spending all our time together. Then it happened again. I missed a period. I was confused because we were using condoms.

But this time I was scared and a little excited at the same time. I thought to myself, "I have a boyfriend that really cares for me" and I thought he would be excited too. I was remembering what he told me about his girlfriend who had an abortion. He was really disappointed she had an abortion. So I was expecting him to say something like "It will be ok. We can do this together."

Instead, when I told him he turned white as a ghost. There was a long pause and he said, "We can't have this baby. I think you need to get an abortion." I told him, "I can't get another abortion." He then said, "You have two choices. Get the abortion and I stay, or have the baby and I leave".

I was in shock. I really didn't want to have another abortion. My heart and mind were in battle. What should I do? I was so scared. Would I be able to find another guy to love me like Tim loved me? Could I take the chance to lose him? I really loved him. I needed him so much. I was scared to be alone again. This time I was more scared of losing Tim than of God and I chose to have a second abortion.

Second Abortion

We got up early in the morning and Tim drove me to the same clinic I went to the first time. This time my emotions were very different. I didn't want to be there because I knew what I was getting ready to go through.

As we sat in the lobby waiting for my name to be called I was hoping that he would say, "Myrtzie, let's leave. We can have this baby." I was sitting there praying for that to happen and then I heard my name called. It made me jump because I was deep in thought -- imagining us having this baby together --- so when I heard my name it interrupted my daydream and I lost all hope.

My heart sank to my feet and I got up and walked to the back to that little counseling room where again they explained the procedure. Tim stayed in the lobby so I was alone as I walked down the hallway to the medical room where the abortion procedure would take place.

As I lay on the table I could feel the tears running down my face. The nurse grabbed my hand and assured me I was going to be ok. Again I felt the suction and knew what was happening. I felt they were not only sucking my baby out, but they were also sucking my soul out. I was never going to be ok again. It was so surreal.

After it was all over, all I could do was cry. Tim put his arm around me and helped me get in the car. On the car ride home it was very quiet, but every now and then he could hear me sniffle. Then he looked over at me and said, "You know, Myrtzie, if you wouldn't have had the abortion, I would have married you". At that moment, I felt a surge of rage come over me. I wanted to scream, but instead I literally turned myself off, just like a light switch. It was better to feel NOTHING than what I wanted to do. I think if I didn't turn myself off, I could have killed him.

The Aftermath

We continued to date, but were very dysfunctional. We fought a lot and after a while fighting became the norm in our relationship. I became an emotional eater and that also caused problems between the two of us. I was just so miserable on the inside I sabotaged our relationship without even knowing what I was doing.

I decided I was going to make sure I wouldn't get pregnant again so I started using a diaphragm. I became pretty confident this was an effective birth control. We continued to work through our issues and it seemed like all was going great. He proposed to me and I accepted. I was very excited that we were going to get married and start a family together.

My life seemed like it was getting better. I had graduated from beauty school and I got my license to become a cosmetologist. Tim was working hard and saving money. We were planning for our wedding. Everything seemed great.

Then one night, while staying at the beach for a few days --- having a good time with some friends -- Tim and I decided to take a walk on the beach and began to talk about some things. He said he was concerned about me gaining some weight and wondered if I would be a good wife for him. We went back and forth with our discussion and finally decided to call off the wedding. I was devastated.

I didn't agree with his concerns. I thought they were easy enough to work through and definitely didn't think they were enough to call off the wedding. Two weeks later, to my surprise I missed my period.

I went and took a pregnancy test and the test came out positive. This time I was scared for just a minute and then I got this strength I never knew I had. I called Tim and told him I wanted to go out to dinner, so he came and picked me up. This time I gave him the ultimatum. I told him, "I took a pregnancy test and it came out positive. I have thought about this a lot and have decided I am going to have this baby with you or without you. You can either marry me or leave me, I don't care, but I am having this baby!"

He chose marriage and we were married two months later. I will never forget our experience at our twelve week checkup. We were scheduled for our first sonogram; we both were excited to see our baby. I was not expecting to see what we saw. Wow! We could see our baby's heartbeat, and then we heard the heartbeat. My heart was overjoyed. Then we saw her ten fingers and ten toes. She was even sucking on her thumb. We were amazed.

I couldn't believe what I was seeing. The abortion clinic told me it was a blob of tissue. They told me it wasn't a baby. But what I was seeing was a baby, our baby. WHAT DID I DO? Flashbacks of both of my abortions came crashing to my mind. My heart was devastated again with regret and shame.

We got married in September. Afterward, our relationship changed for the better. He did explain that when he called off our wedding that day on the beach, it was just last minute jitters. He said he had cold feet and he was scared of making that final commitment and had never stopped loving me. That made me feel better and more secure in our relationship. We both were enjoying the anticipation of our baby.

Motherhood

Then the most amazing day happened, my daughter was born. I will never forget the love I experienced when the doctor put my daughter on my chest. All the pain I was in from the C-section didn't matter. After everybody left I held her in my arms in amazement. We counted all her little fingers and toes. At that moment my life changed.

She inspired me to want more. I wanted the world for her. I made a commitment to God to change. I wanted to be the best mother that I could be and Tim wanted to be the best father he could be. We made a decision to be better together.

Then in 1988 I gave birth to my second daughter and I was in Mommy Heaven. I loved being a mother. My entire life revolved around my children. We were dealing with the everyday struggles of being new parents, balancing schedules and being a wife and mother. Then we had our third daughter in 1990.

Now we were proud parents of three daughters. Life got so busy and it became more difficult to balance life. And every time I would look at my daughters who I loved so much I thought about the two that I had aborted. I would think of all the opportunities in their lives that I missed out on. I began to get depressed and didn't know why.

I was juggling between children, my home day care business and being involved with my church and my kid's school. I felt I had to overcompensate. I had to be a good mom and a good church-goer. Deep down, I think I was trying to earn my way back into God's grace.

Because of what I had done in the past, my children were a constant reminder to me of all that I had missed by aborting my other children. As a result, I began to struggle with depression. I noticed Tim and I began fighting more often, and once again I was sabotaging our relationship. Our marriage at this point was hanging on a thread. He thought everything was ok, but I felt like I was dying on the inside.

Then one evening I was at a teachers' meeting at our church when the topic of abortion came up. This conversation made me very uncomfortable, but I spoke up once and said "You never know what the girl might be going through." Then I just sat silent listening to the conversation. My heart started to beat really fast. My hands started to sweat. My skin started to turn red and I just had to get out of there. So I got up and went outside for a while. Then I saw another teacher come out.

She happened to be the mother of one of my students. We were standing outside talking when -- out of the blue --- I began to cry and tell her I had two abortions. Then she began to cry and told me she had two abortions as well. I had never told anyone about that before. I was surprised that it even came out of my mouth. That's how I knew it must have been a God thing.

That night I went home and was sitting out in my front yard with my husband, swinging on our swing together. I remember him asking me why I was so quiet. I began to cry and said to him, "I am going to Hell for what I have done".

He asked me, "What do you mean?" and I explained to him, "I am the one who had two abortions. I am the one going to hell." I just sat there and cried. How could God forgive me for that? I cried to him saying, "I give up. How can I be a good mother or a good wife? Look what I have done! I took my two children's lives away. I don't deserve to go to Heaven."

I remember feeling this overwhelming fear that I had lost my salvation. I didn't know how to get it back. Everything I tried didn't work. I felt like I would take one step forward and two steps back. I knew my way wasn't working and I felt like I was failing at everything that mattered in my life --- as a wife and mother. I guess you could say I hit rock bottom.

The next morning we received the Florida Catholic and Tim read an article in it about a Post Abortion Recovery group called First Steps, which was located at the First Life Center for Pregnancy. Tim told me about it and encouraged me to go to it. He said, "Maybe this will help you feel better." I agreed and called the other teacher. We decided to go the group together.

First Steps: A Biblical Study for Abortion Recovery

The first night it was very hard to go because I didn't know what to expect, but I was also excited at the same time because I didn't even know anything like this group existed. The Recovery Group --- or this Pregnancy Center I should say --- was associated with a church. I was scared of being judged and rejected. But I was accepted with open arms. They greeted us with a hug and were very hospitable.

The atmosphere was pleasant and they made me feel very safe to share. There was a leader and a co-leader and about five other women besides my friend and myself. We went around the circle sharing what prompted us to attend this group. It was very easy to open up and I remember how good it felt to share, but what felt even better was hearing the other girls share. There were a lot of similarities and for the first time I didn't feel so alone.

On my way home, I remember thinking how much better I felt and couldn't imagine what else the group could cover, but the eleven week Bible Study had many more issues to cover and every week I learned something new and was able to give God a little more of myself each time. My experience turned out to be a journey of healing, which felt like a roller coaster ride at times. Sometimes the memories were very painful and sometimes it was great to learn and experience God's Word coming alive in my life. It was so amazing. I had often heard the Word of God called the Living Word, but I never truly understood what it meant until this Bible Study. His Word literally came to life and grabbed me. For example in Psalm 51 (NIV):

"¹ Have mercy on me, O God, according to your unfailing love; according to your great compassion blot out my transgressions. ² Wash away all my iniquity and cleanse me from my sin.

³ For I know my transgressions, and my sin is always before me. ⁴ Against you, you only, have I sinned and done what is evil in your sight; so you are right in your verdict and justified when you judge. ⁵ Surely I was sinful at birth, sinful from the time my mother conceived me. ⁶ Yet you desired faithfulness even in the womb; you taught me wisdom in that secret place.

⁷ Cleanse me with hyssop, and I will be clean; wash me, and I will be whiter than snow ⁸ let me hear joy and gladness; let the bones you have crushed rejoice. ⁹ Hide your face from my sins and blot out all my iniquity.

¹⁰ Create in me a pure heart, O God, and renew a steadfast spirit within me. ¹¹ Do not cast me from your presence or take your Holy Spirit from me. ¹² Restore to me the joy of your salvation and grant me a willing spirit, to sustain me.

¹³ Then I will teach transgressors your ways, so that sinners will turn back to you. ¹⁴ Deliver me from the guilt of bloodshed, O God, you who are God my Savior, and my tongue will sing of your righteousness. ¹⁵ Open my lips, Lord, and my mouth will declare your praise. ¹⁶ You do not delight in sacrifice, or I would bring it; you do not take pleasure in burnt offerings. ¹⁷ My sacrifice, O God, is a broken spirit; a broken and contrite heart you, God, will not despise.

¹⁸ May it please you to prosper Zion, to build up the walls of Jerusalem. ¹⁹ Then you will delight in the sacrifices of the righteous, in burnt offerings offered whole; then bulls will be offered on your altar."

In the reference, the writer David was feeling guilty because he had committed adultery with a woman named Bathsheba and had her husband killed. He knew his actions had hurt many people. He knew God had forgiven him, as no sin is too great for God to forgive, but he was still living with the consequences. God forgives our sins, but does not take our consequences away. David's family was never the same after what he did, just like my life was changed after my two abortions.

I can remember feeling this way. Every time I would try to get closer to God or become a better person, my sin was forever before me. It was like getting slapped in the face or hitting a brick wall. I would hear Satan's lies…"Myrtzie you're not good enough. Myrtzie you don't deserve to have God love you."

In verse seven, the Hyssop branch is what the Israelites in Egypt used to rub lamb's blood over their doors to keep them safe from death. This is what David is calling out to God for --- for cleansing and to be set free from captivity.

As we studied this, I thought back on that night when I was sitting with my husband on our swing explaining to him I was going to Hell because I thought God couldn't forgive me for murder. I truly thought I had lost my salvation. When I read about David asking God to renew his spirit and restore the joy of his salvation, I wanted the same restoration. I began to call out to God as David did. Ask God to create a pure heart and spirit in you. He is waiting for you to call out to Him.

Verses 13-17 explain exactly how I felt --- knowing God had forgiven me and I had experienced His mercy. I wanted to shout it from the mountain tops. Then I wanted God to help me share that truth with other men and women who were hurting. Having experienced God's Word come alive, He restored my relationship with Him. He tore down my brick wall brick by brick.

God does not delight in sacrifice or burnt offering anymore. In the Old Testament the larger the sin the larger animal needed for a sacrifice. But after Jesus was crucified on the cross as the final sacrifice for ALL of our sins, God no longer wanted animal sacrifice from us. Now all He wants is our broken hearts and broken spirits to be given to Him.

When I first came to the First Steps Bible Study I was just like Humpty Dumpty. I was a broken person and no one could put me back together again. It wasn't until I gave my brokenness to God and chose to believe God's truths that God put me back together again and restored me and my relationship with Him. Through God's Scripture and the segment of the group called Sharing Time, I learned how to accept God's forgiveness, His mercy and His grace, which brought restoration to my life. As a result, I rededicated my life to Christ. As much as my two abortions were a negative life changing experience, my rededication changed my life for the better. God saved my marriage and helped me to become a better mother, daughter and friend. Completing the Bible Study brought me closer to Christ, changed my life and gave me hope for my future. Now instead of walking with my head held low in shame I can walk with my head held high in righteousness.

> *"But you, Lord, are a shield around me, my glory, the One who lifts my head high." Psalm 3:3*

Now God has laid it upon my heart to help other women to choose life for their babies. However, for the ones who still choose to abort, I want to help them find God's forgiveness, Grace and Mercy. God is waiting to do what Isaiah 61:2-3 says:

> *"To comfort all who mourn, To console those who mourn in Zion, To give them Beauty for Ashes, the oil of joy for mourn ing, The garment of praise for the spirit of heaviness."*

He wants to bring peace back into your life. He wants to bring you back to emotional and spiritual wellness.

My prayer for you is that First Steps Bible Study and the journaling process will help you as much as it has helped me. First Steps will lead you to God's Word and your healing will come from God your Father in Heaven.

YOUR FIRST STEP

After reading the stories of these courageous women, were you able to see how the aftermath of an abortion will affect you, regardless of whether you were the person who had the abortion or the person who helped either in the decision making process or by driving them to the abortion clinic. No matter how we try to justify abortion, the choice to abort was against God's will. This is why it affects us emotionally and spiritually.

I found out the hard way God gave us boundaries because He loves us. For example, picture Jesus as a Shepherd and He has all of the sheep in a wooden fence. The fence is there to protect the sheep from the wolf who is waiting to attack them. But as soon as a lamb escapes through the fence he is wide open for the wolf to attack. It is like that for us. As soon as we step outside of God's boundaries we are wide open for Satan's attack. For so many years I believed Satan's lies. In John 8:42-45 it says:

"Jesus said to them, "If God were your Father, you would love Me, for I proceeded forth and have come from God, for I have not even come on My own initiative, but He sent Me. Why do you not understand what I am saying? It is because you cannot hear My word. You are of your father the devil, and you want to do the desires of your father. He was a murderer from the beginning, and does not stand in the truth because there is no truth in him. Whenever he speaks a lie, he speaks from his own nature, for he is a liar and the father of lies. But because I speak the truth, you do not believe Me." (NASB)

How many years have you believed Satan's lies? Lies such as:

> *"You are not good enough for God. God can't forgive you. Why should He? You have had several abortions. You don't deserve a good life. You need to be punished a little more."*

Those are ALL lies. Those lies have kept you in bondage for a long time. It is time for you to reveal the lies of Satan and replace them with God's TRUTH.

Imagine yourself in a dark box. All you can see is darkness and you can feel the heaviness of your sins all around you. Then God speaks the truth from His Word and that truth punctures a small pin hole of light. Then He reveals some more truth like Proverbs 30:5 *"Every Word of God is flawless; He is a shield to those who take refuge in Him."* And 1 John 4:9-10 *"This is how God showed His love among us: He sent His one and only Son into the world that we might live through Him. This is love: not that we loved God, but that He loved us and sent His Son as an atoning sacrifice for our sins."*

God will keep revealing His truth and before you know the darkness is gone, your burden has been lifted and you have been set free from your sin.

God loves you right now ---right where you are at in your life --- mistakes and all. He is waiting for you to come to Him. He is ready for you to lay your burden at the foot of His Cross. He is ready to carry you on your own Journey of Healing. Trust in Him and take your first step towards healing and hope.

Allow the Word of God to come into your life and grab you, and embrace you with truth and love. Take that first step and experience the Word. It will be your balm of Gilead.

So Shall My word be that goes out from
my mouth; it shall NOT RETURN to me
Empty, but it shall accom that which
I Purpose and Shall SUCCEE
in the th to Which I sent
IT." So s my be that goes
Out from mouth it shall not
Return e PURP but it shall
accomplish which I
purpose and thing for which
Susan Granville Cray

It Embraces You!

You see my beloved when you choose to believe God's truth and accept Him into your life as your Lord and Savior, you get adopted into the Royal Family of God. He becomes your King of Kings and you become his Princess. You become a daughter of a King! All you have to do is admit that you are a sinner.

We are all sinners. Romans 3:23 *"For all have sinned and fall short of the glory of God."* When we sin it can lead to death. Romans 6:23 says *"For the wages of sin is death."* When we sin it separates us from Christ. But the good news is that God sent His only son Jesus Christ to die for you.

Romans 5:8 says *"But God demonstrates His own love toward us, in that while we were still sinners, Christ died for us."* My beloved Jesus took all the punishment for us so we wouldn't have to be punished. We can be saved through your faith in Jesus Christ.

Ephesians 2:8-9 says, *"For by grace (undeserved favor) you have been saved and that not of yourselves; it is the gift of God, not of works, lest anyone should boast."* You see you can't earn your way to Heaven. You are not good enough. By going to church every Sunday, or just by being a good person, you do not deserve to be saved to go to Heaven. It is only by God's grace and because Jesus was sacrificed so we could be forgiven. You have to accept God's grace and truth and pray to Him. Here's a sample prayer:

Lord, I am a sinner. I chose to have an abortion(s). I killed my baby/babies that already had a plan and a purpose for their lives. I missed out on opportunities to love them and parent them. Lord I will never get to hold them here on earth. I will not get to see them grow. I am so sorry for not having the courage to choose life. I am sorry for hurting You. I never realized how many lives I hurt by my choice. Please forgive me. I need You as my Lord and Savior. I need You to come into my life. Please Lord fill my heart with Your Holy Spirit. I know that you died for my sins and I am so grateful that you have forgiven me. Amen.

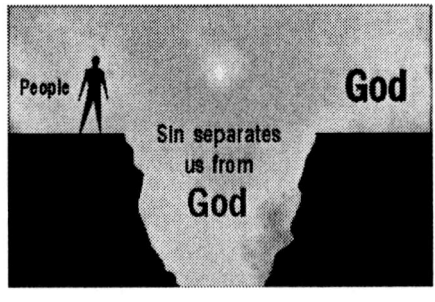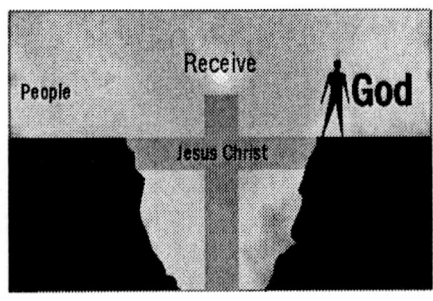

Now choose to walk with your head held high in righteousness and accept God's TRUTH that you have been forgiven and set free from all blood guilt, shame and regret. Now you are a princess… a Daughter of a King!

My Daughter, My Princess

I Am the King of King's and Lord of Lords
I Am the Beginning and the End
I Am the great physician of the world
Your heart is MINE to mend
Victory is yours to claim
Through my Son up on the cross
To take away your shame and guilt
Of the little one's you've lost
The enemy will try to keep you down
And fill your heart with grief
But by My grace you are forgiven
If you choose freely to believe
You are the daughter of a King
Stand proud and use your voice
Dance my precious princess
For it's time that you rejoice
I Am the King of Kings and Lord of Lords
And you belong to Me
No longer shall you walk in shame
My Son has set you free.

Written By: Laurie Maring

I pray you will have courage and take your first step to find healing and hope by reaching out to a Post Abortion healing study that will help you face the many emotions you have experienced in the aftermath of abortion. Even though you might have prayed to receive Jesus and He has forgiven you, I encourage you to start your journey of healing to deal with the symptoms of Post Abortion and find closure to this chapter in your life. My prayers are with you.

BIBLE STUDIES FOR
ABORTION RECOVERY

First Life Center Pregnancy
First Steps to Abortion Recovery
3125 Bruton Blvd. Suite B
Orlando, Fl 32805
Tele: 407-514-4520
Email: Info@FirstStepsJourneytoHealing.com

To find a Recovery group close to you call:

National Helpline for Abortion Recovery
1-866-482-LIFE
24/7 Confidential Care
Nationalhelpline.org

ABOUT THE AUTHOR

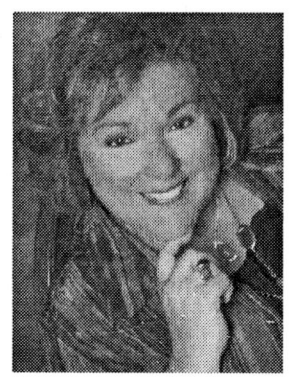 The Program Coordinator of First Life Center for Pregnancy, a ministry of First Baptist Orlando, Author and Teacher, Myrtzie Levell experienced her personal journey to healing and experienced God's Redemption through First Steps in 1994. Since that time, she has had a calling and passion to serve God in the area of Post Abortion Recovery. Through First Steps, Myrtzie has ministered to hundreds of women and men, helping those who are considering abortion choose life, and ministering God's healing power to those who have been wounded by the choice of abortion. She also trains others who share her passion and calling. "I am privileged and humbled to walk alongside men and women who have been hurt by abortion," says Levell.

Myrtzie is a mother to three amazing daughters, Jennifer, Crystal and Sharon and grandmother of four: Jordan, Jay, Landon and Scarlet. She also has two precious children, Alicia and Thomas, whom she looks forward to holding one day when she joins them in Heaven. Myrtzie resides in Orlando, Florida with her husband and best friend of 28 years, Tim Levell.

For more info, media inquiries or to invite Myrtzie to your event, visit *www.MyrtzieLevell.com*.